DEDICATION

In Memory...

Geoff Flowers	Mother, Kathryn Flowers James
Whitt Keyes	Mother, Kathy Keyes
Megan & Tyler Ray	Father, Larry C. Ray Baby Brother, Nathan Nicholson
Jason Hite	Mother, Gloria J. Hite
David Levine	Brother, Phillip James Garner Friend, Baby Kenny Mittlestadt
Kari Deakins	Twin Sister, Shari Anne Deakins
Daniel Navarro	Friends, Joe Robles Victor Alverez Salvador Diaz Luis Vasquez

In Honor...

Blanca Martinez	Parents, Mr. & Mrs. Conrado Martinez

Acknowledgments

I want to thank my school superintendent, Tom Davenport, assistant superintendent, Dawn Angrove, and principals Pat Taliaferro, Ralph Funk, and Rod Southard. I appreciate good friends, Cheryl Hochstetler and Kathy Helm, for their support and encouragement. A big thank you goes to Shaheda Bawa for her information on Muslim traditions, Laura Sweeden on Catholic traditions, and Cyndi A. Villarreal on Jewish traditions. I want to thank my kids, Mike and Michelle, for sharing their wonderful teenage years with me. My husband, Malcom, I thank for his patience and for being there through each phase of this book.

Janet N. Tyson

Table of Contents

INTRODUCTION

A person's life is like a web. All of the parts are interconnected. When there is a break in the structure, the entire web must be reconstructed and healed. Eventually, if the healing has taken a positive course that section of the web will be rewoven into a new, healthy web. This is symbolic of the reinvestment of life. The other parts of the web still have part of the old that was lost, but it has changed, and continues to live. The web concept is also symbolic of the fragility of our lives and the significance of each person that we meet (1).

When I started working with grieving teens in Lake Dallas, Texas, I had no plan to help them write a book. Actually, the idea originated during a grief support group meeting when everyone described how they were coping by writing about their losses. The techniques and methods were different, but writing helped them remember and work through their feelings in order to make it through one more day. These students wanted to help other grieving teens cope by sharing what they had written.

The students in the grief group asked me to write a counselor's perspective on teenage grief for their book. For me, the best method involved writing about the relationship I had with each one of them, the strategies that were used, and recommended guidelines for facilitating grief. The results of our efforts read like a narrative.

In the spring of 1994, our school lost a student who was killed in a car accident. Methods are included in this book that were used to help our teens and teachers deal with losing a student.

Common Threads of Teenage Grief helps teens and the people who love them work through the grieving process. Teens learn how to deal with their pain and memories and move on with their lives. Parents learn what their children need and want from them. This book also gives school counselors, preachers, friends, and families successful methods used to help teens recover.

We hope you find the peace you are seeking by reading this book.

1

Stuff for Teenagers

TEENS ARE UNIQUE

The teenage years can be exciting but also somewhat frightening at times. You will experience more physical and sexual changes, mental and emotional upheaval, and make more social choices in your life than at any other time since you were born. During the teenage years, most people try to gain independence by emotionally pulling away from their parents and establishing their own identities (2). Friends take on an important role and a majority of your time is spent with them. However, your home and your emotional ties to the people in it remain strong.

These years also can be confusing and contradictory for you. Although teens want to appear in control and "cool," most of you are sensitive to criticism, possess a strong sense of fairness, ask questions about moral and ethical issues, and reflect about life. You may not always want it, but you often need support and structure. It is common for teens to begin hiding their problems or worry from their parents.

Life Happens

Things happen to the people you know and love that are out of your control. They just happen. Parents, siblings, or friends become ill or die in accidents. Teen friends often make risky choices and don't always consider the consequences.

Accidents are the number one cause of teenage death for 15 to 24 year olds. Homicides and suicides are the second and third causes, respectively, of death for 15 to 24 year olds. In 1995, 76.5 percent of teenage accidental deaths were due to car accidents (3). Many young drivers do not see danger in the risks they are taking. Instead some use their driving to assert their independence, express anger and frustration, and gain acceptance of peers by driving too fast, being aggressive, and taking chances (4).

In 1995 there were 6,827 teenage deaths in the U.S. from homicides. Many teenagers have friends who become victims of gang violence. There are approximately 665,000 gang members in the United States (5). According to Detective Sam Schiller of The Dallas Police Gang Unit, "Although there are variances from area to area, gangs exist in communities throughout the United States. Most teenagers join in order to belong to a group and to be recognized. In the last 10 years, gangs have spread to middle-class neighborhoods as a result of individual members moving there. Our efforts continue to reach 'fringe' members and show them there is a better way of life without the gang."

Suicide among young people historically is a serious problem. In 1995, 5,350 people, 15 to 24 years-old, killed themselves (6). Teenagers have big stressors like drug abuse, teen pregnancy, AIDS, divorced parents, and violence in schools. They also have to deal with every day problems, such as arguments with family or friends, peer pressure, relationship issues, and school performance. All of these stressful situations put teenagers at risk for depression which may lead to suicide. Studies have shown that loss of a family member, parental alcohol use, experiencing abuse or neglect, and arguing with parents are the main reasons teenagers attempt and complete suicide (7).

HOW DO MOST PEOPLE HANDLE GRIEF ?

Losing someone you love hurts. The shock of hearing about the death can be intense and your reactions depend upon your emotional investment in the relationship with the person you lost.

Some people want to escape the pain of death by not dealing with it. Others think showing emotion like crying, proves weakness. Therefore, they try to be stoic and hide their true feelings.

Role models, like pro athletes, movie stars, and political figures, set standards that others try to follow. Unfortunately, some role models stifle their emotions after losing a loved one because they do not want to appear weak. Their behavior sends the wrong message. If you choose to ignore your pain of loss, chances are you will have to deal with it later. Most counselors encourage people to allow themselves to feel their grief, cry, and share--talk about it. It usually helps to attend the person's funeral to say good-bye.

Societies and the major religions in those societies help determine how people feel about death. In the United States there is a decline of rituals and traditions that help people recover from losing a loved one. Many people do not know what to expect and wonder if their experiences are normal. Actually, funerals, wakes, and mourning rites help people confront their grief and eventually heal.

In our society, there are many cultural and ethnic groups with various religious beliefs. These groups have their own traditions and ways of dealing with death and dying. Diversity among groups sometimes makes it difficult to understand the grieving behavior of others (8, 9). To help you understand your own and others' religious traditions, read the section on funeral traditions on pages 107-108.

COMPLICATED GRIEVING

Progression through grief may be interrupted by behavior that complicates and delays the healing. These unhealthy reactions block, prolong, or mask grief. During this time, the person with a loss may be unable to function or concentrate on simple every day tasks. Physical or mental problems may develop as a result of the stress.

Circumstances that Complicate Grieving (10, 11)

* *Suppressed Grief:* Some people feel the pain of losing someone is more than they can endure, therefore, they suppress their grief by staying very busy or doing other things to ignore their pain. Others try to dull their feelings by abusing alcohol or other drugs. Unfortunately, addictions can develop from the drug abuse, which causes even more problems. Suppressing grief by using these different methods kills release of emotions and blocks recovery from grief.

* *Lack of Support:* Another circumstance that complicates grieving is lack of support. Few people may be available or willing to offer comfort and support to the person suffering a loss. Without a friendly environment that encourages grieving, a person's healing is often delayed. Sometimes you need someone to help you make decisions and other times just being there for you is enough.

* *Multiple Losses:* Circumstances are also complicated if you recently had to deal with divorce, death, or other loss of someone close. Previous deaths or losses may make the current situation overwhelming. Some of these losses may not thoroughly be resolved by the survivor and they may add to the confusion. Losses that occur close together complicate grieving and often lead to mental or physical problems.

Traumatic or Unexpected Death: Death that is sudden, like a natural disaster, an accident, suicide, or death due to violence, gives you little time to prepare mentally or emotionally. Due to the shock and related stress, those left behind may be unable to develop coping strategies.

Health Status: Poor mental or physical health can weaken your ability to heal. Many times health problems come as a result of the loss. Under these circumstances, chronic depression becomes a concern and usually involves withdrawing from society and personal activities (9).

Extremely Close Relationship With Person Who Is Gone: When an especially close or dependent relationship existed, you may not heal as quickly. By not accepting the loss, you hold onto the loved one a little longer and delay taking independent action (10). Carried to an extreme, this could be a problem.

WHAT ARE COMMON THREADS OF TEENAGE GRIEF?

When someone dies they care about, teenagers share many similar grief reactions. However, it is not always easy to identify these common threads in teens because they are very good at hiding their true feelings. With knowledge and understanding, people who care can help teenagers heal and recover from grief. Adults may also experience many of these same reactions but often handle them differently because of more life experience and maturity.

Common Threads (11, 12, 13, 14)

Struggle With Guilt: Teenagers struggle with guilt because of past efforts to be independent and achieve a life style separate from their families. Teens feel guilty for the way they acted or for harsh words they said or endearing words they did not say. A teenager can actually feel responsible for their loved one's death and think that somehow he or she could have prevented it.

   * *Devastated by "Good-byes":* Teens who missed an opportunity to say good-bye, live with the reality of knowing they will never have another chance. For those teenagers who said "good-bye," it remains a painfully vivid memory.

   * *Face Grief Alone:* Except when teens have lost a mutual friend and they come together and bond, many teens face their grief alone. When they lose a parent or sibling, teen friends do not always come around because they feel uncomfortable and do not know what to say. In this circumstance, grieving teens learn *not* to talk about their losses because it makes their friends feel uneasy. At home, many surviving family members also are dealing with grief and are incapable of helping their grieving children.

   * *Try to Be Strong for Family:* Commonly, teenagers assume the role of caretaker of family members while denying their own emotions. They often feel they must remain strong and stoic for their family. These young people may appear to be coping with the death when they are not.

   * *Escape for Older Teens:* Teenagers, who have access to a car, manage to leave home and stay busy with school activities and jobs. This type of behavior allows them to deny or avoid the loss and may put them at risk for long term resolution. This type of response does not always have negative results. However, escaping can delay the healing process.

* *Isolation for Younger Teens:* Teenagers, 13 to 15 years old, are less independent than older teens. They spend more time at home with their families and are less involved with outside activities. Studies show these young teens have a tendency to be more withdrawn and may become preoccupied and attached to their lost parent, other family member, or friend (12).

* *Identify Future Losses:* Like adults, young people recognize the fact there will be more losses related to the present death. Their deceased friend or family member will not share their futures. Special occasions like graduations, weddings, and births will be celebrated without their loved ones.

* *Form Emotional Bond With Lost Sibling:* When there is a death of a brother or sister, a bond is created with the lost sibling and involves many dimensions. The surviving sibling continues to bond with the lost sibling through shared past experiences, present every day thoughts, or future anticipation of reuniting after this life on earth. The survivor may ask the deceased sibling to "guide and help me."

* *Experience Dysfunctions:* Sleep disturbances, depression, and inability to concentrate at school are common for the grieving teenager. Some teens also experience behavioral problems after a loss.

Anger is Natural

The release of anger is the result of frustration felt when you realize that no matter what you do, nothing will change the fact that your loved one is dead. Usually the death is not expected, therefore, you may perceive it as unfair. Being angry gives you a sense of power which makes you feel in control. This feeling counteracts your sense of fright and helplessness (15). When you feel anger, you may need to release it. Be careful not to harm property, anyone else, or yourself. Suggested ways to deal with anger constructively are:

- Hit a mattress with a tennis racket, bat, or shoe;
- Tear newspapers or magazines into shreds and throw it away;
- Smash ice cubes with a hammer; throw cubes outside;
- Punch a pillow; pound nails with a hammer;
- Yell in the shower or with loud music playing;
- Write bad words on a piece of paper, wad it up and throw it away;
- Describe the anger on a piece of paper, then stomp on the paper;
- Draw your interpretation of anger and throw away;
- Run or jog; play your favorite sport;
- Throw a basketball at a hoop;
- Hit a tennis ball on a backboard;
- Throw a sponge in the shower;
- Write an angry letter, wad it up, and throw away;
- Do house chores that require large amounts of energy like mopping, mowing, or raking leaves;
- Practice relaxation techniques, blow out tension and anger. Breathe in peace and calm.

Although in gang life it is common to seek revenge for a senseless killing, past gang members admit the acts of revenge only temporarily made the pain of loss go away. It didn't make it stay away and sometimes caused more grief to follow (5).

HOW CAN YOU WORK THROUGH GRIEF?

You can help yourself heal and grow through the grief process. The following two lists may help you heal.

Suggestions to Help You Get
Through the First Difficult Days

- Recognize and feel your pain and cry.

- Describe your pain and list five fears to someone at home like your parent, older sibling, cousin, aunt, uncle or clergy.

- Talk to your school counselor.

- Lean on your friends, let them do for you.

- Start a daily journal so you can express your feelings.

- Make a scrapbook or picture album to commemorate the person you lost.

- Write a poem or letter to the person you lost.

- Consider planting a tree in your yard or community for a living memorial.

- Rely on your strength and courage.

- Remember that each day is a new beginning.

- Join a teenage grief group.

- Read a book on grief and loss.

Helping Yourself in Times of Grief

(c) 1989 Donna O'Toole, M.A.
Reproduced from *Growing Through Grief: A K-12 Curriculum to Help Young People Through All Kinds of Loss*

Here are some lanterns to light the path and guide you on your journey through grief. They are guidelines written by pathfinders who have traveled through grief before you.

1. Seek and Accept Support.
You need acceptance and caring throughout grief. If you lack support, make finding it your first goal. Start with family, friends, or clergy...or call a local counseling agency or school counselor for advice.

2. Accept Your Grief.
Time alone may not heal grief. To work through it, you must accept and deal with it. Remember it is a natural healing process. Roll with its tides.

3. Find Models.
You may need evidence that survival and growth are possible. Look for someone who can give you this hope. Books and support groups may be good places to begin.

4. Learn About Grief.
Many people declare, "I found out I'm not crazy...I'm grieving." Understanding grief can make it safer and more predictable.

5. Express It.
Without expression, grief can leave you frozen and stoic. Find someone who can listen to your story--again and again. You may also want to express it privately...through music, art, poetry or a journal.

6. Accept Your Feelings.
Grief has many feelings...some very intense. Accept them and they will help you learn about yourself and the meaning of your loss. Lock them up inside you and you will lock away parts of yourself.

7. Pace Yourself.
Grief takes energy. You may tire easily. A slower pace alternated with periods of diversion and mild exercise will maximize healing. So will good nutrition; eat 3 times per day.

8. Involve Yourself in Work or Meaningful Activity.
It can help you maintain direction, control and purpose, and occupy your mind.

9. Don't Be Afraid to Have Fun.
Laughter IS good medicine. Allow yourself opportunities for diversion and freshness. Children and pets are great providers of healing. Nurture a friendship with someone who can help you play.

10. Hitch Your Wagon to a Star.
Faith is not the absence of fear, but the willingness to go on when fear is present. Healing will come eventually.

WHAT IS IT LIKE TO FEEL BETTER?

Grief seems endless, but eventually you reach a point where your feelings of loss are not as intense as they once were. The anger, guilt, and regret diminish and so do unexpected emotions of grief once triggered by everyday incidents. For the first time, loss is no longer the focal point of your life and you appear to be in control.

Recovery from a loss, does not mean that you forget your loved one or that you will resume life exactly as it was before the death. You have been deeply hurt and the "emotional scar tissue" will ache from time to time (16). Your life will never be exactly the same again, but you gain strength from knowing you have worked through such intense grief.

People who reach this point and feel better after a loss, often change in positive ways. You may develop an empathy and desire to help others with losses. Life has new meaning and you may develop different perspectives and fresh attitudes toward your future. You may rededicate yourself to your studies or work or hobbies. Now, you can identify your successes and move forward.

2
Grieving & Growing

As a school counselor, my interest in helping students deal with grief began when a seventh-grade student, I will call Anna, lost her twin sister, Mary, in an accident. Mary's death was unexpected and left the family in shock. Anna was devastated. It affected her physically, mentally, and emotionally. The last two months of school that year, she merely went through the motions to finish.

Three months later after summer break, Anna was continuing to have a difficult time. At home, her parents were making decisions regarding her sister's photographs and personal items. The painful chore affected the whole family. Wishing that Mary had not died, Anna wanted everything to remain exactly the same.

At school there also were constant reminders of her loss: pictures in yearbooks, her sister's old locker and friends. She became upset about comments someone made about sisters and other random topics discussed in class. Often she would be sitting in class concentrating and without warning, an overwhelming emotion would engulf her.

Anna asked to talk to me. She talked at length about her sister. She did the talking, and I occasionally asked questions. I encouraged her to remember, recognize, and feel, not deny her memories. After visiting with her twice a week for four weeks, she began to remember and describe funny incidents with her sister. They were wonderful stories, and together we laughed at those memories. She also expressed frustration about some things her sister had done. This indicated she had made some progress toward working through her grief.

In October of that same year, a sixth-grade teacher requested I visit with Whitt, a student whose mother died after a long illness. The first time I met him, Whitt was very attentive but also very quiet. The appointment was the teacher's idea, not his, and he was not ready to talk. I explained to him what to expect regarding his feelings of loss and challenges he could expect in the days ahead. I let him know I would be available if he needed to visit with me again. When he left my office, I did not know if I would ever see him again. Six weeks after his mother's death, Whitt came and asked if he could visit. The shock of his mother's death had subsided and in his current mental state he was unable to concentrate or finish his school work. Thoughts of his mother kept creeping into his head. Whitt wanted help.

Although I knew there was some risk in combining sessions, after visiting with Whitt for a month, I asked if he would like to meet with Anna. Anna and Whitt did not know each other, they attended different schools, and Whitt was two years younger. Yet, grief, the common ingredient existed. Both had processed through some grief and they were at the same stage of recovery.

ANNA AND WHITT MEET

From the beginning, the combined sessions were successful. Anna and Whitt understood each other's grief. In fact, dialogue was so immediate and continuous that I soon became an interested observer. One would say, "Did you...?" or, "Would they...?" The other one would respond quickly with, "Yea, and...!" The time spent with these two teenagers (Whitt became 13 this year) gave me great insight into the needs of grieving teens.

Because music has special meaning to individuals dealing with grief, one topic these teenagers discussed was music. They identified with songs that expressed their feelings or reminded them of their losses. The process helped them get in touch with their feelings and appeared to have a positive affect. The tough time came right before Thanksgiving. Department stores and malls were playing holiday music for Christmas shoppers. The two were not prepared for the impact that such special music would have on them. How could anyone listen to music and enjoy themselves when this time of the year was so painful for them? Both avoided cheerful crowds throughout Thanksgiving and Christmas breaks.

Holidays are difficult especially for someone in grief, and I tried to prepare them. Both needed to be with family members who were willing to explore new holiday activities the teens could look forward to. It appeared both teens were going to be with many close family members who would feel comfortable enough to share conversation about the deceased, but would encourage a great deal of activity.

After the Christmas holidays both teens showed signs of depression. They had unpredictable emotional swings, trouble concentrating on simple tasks, general overall feelings of being tired most of the time, and a desire to be alone. Anna was having problems with her appetite and appeared to be losing weight. Later, she had many colds, flu, and illnesses. Our combined sessions continued. They talked a great deal and worked hard to process through the feelings of each stage of grief they experienced.

Observing The First Year Anniversary

Soon, the dreaded first year anniversary of Anna's sister's death was only two months away. All three of us knew this would be a difficult time. However, we would be there to support her and get her through that day. As time passed, we began making plans for that special day. The teenagers decided they wanted to plant two trees in front of our school as a memorial for her sister and his mother.

I will never forget Anna's and Whitt's reactions when I said, "You can tie blue ribbons around each tree!" Whitt abruptly asked, "Why blue ribbons?" I answered, "To signify life. The sky is blue, birds fly free in the sky." He said, "But my mother's favorite color was red!" Anna quickly said, "And my sister's favorite color was green!" The ribbon colors were decided that fast.

Two months passed quickly and on the anniversary of Mary's death, Anna and Whitt, accompanied by their best friends, came to my office after the first bell of the day. We went outside to the front of the school building and watched as a school district employee dug two deep holes six feet apart. Whitt's dad drove up in his car at this time, but Whitt requested he not stay. Whitt wanted to keep this a special event between himself and his mother. His dad understood and left.

When the employee finished planting the trees, he collected his tools and disappeared. Whitt took the red ribbon and along with his friend, tied a bow around the trunk of one tree. With the help of her friend, Anna tied a green ribbon on the second tree. Then, without saying a word, Whitt's friend stood by him and placed his hand on Whitt's shoulder. Anna's friend stood by her and did the same. We stood between the trees as I read a poem that had been the sister's favorite. Then, we stood in silence with bowed heads. After a minute or so, I invited the four teenagers to my office for cake. The solemn mood was respectful and almost cheerful. I wanted to allow time for the young people to visit together without me. I quickly found busy work in the front office.

After fifteen minutes, I returned to my office where the four teenagers were finishing their cake. The two friends, who had been thoughtful and supportive all morning, returned to their classes. Anna and Whitt followed in a few minutes. If this were an event among family or friends, not on a school day, it would have been appropriate to go out for lunch or some other special activity.

Anna thanked Whitt and me for giving her a memorable morning and making something good out of a bad situation. If it had not been for our carefully planned activities, she would have stayed home from school.

Each day, our attention was drawn by the two trees with their red and green ribbons blowing in the breeze. "They look really good there, don't they!" "How big will they get?" "Who waters the trees around here?"

I warned them the ribbons probably would not last long because students waited for school buses near the trees. I was sure the ribbons would disappear soon in such a high traffic area and I was concerned about the teens' reactions. To my surprise, the bright fabric remained untouched for three months. The last week of school these two teenagers who had shared so much untied the ribbons and carefully placed them in manila envelopes to take home.

Taking Care of the Trees

That following summer was hot and dry. Every time I drove somewhere, I detoured by the school to check on the trees. Finally, my husband and I decided we must water the trees or they would die. We could not find a hydrant, so we hauled buckets of water for five weeks. The trees survived a hostile Texas summer.

Recovery for Whitt

Whitt played baseball that hot summer and Anna was busy with relatives and friends. When school started in the fall, although he never expressed it, I could tell Whitt missed visiting with Anna who was now attending high school. After a close relationship for two years, I missed her too.

That year was difficult for Whitt. I continued to visit with him once a week. Many times when we were together, he worked on a project for his grief support group we started that year. I think that helped him more than anything else he could have done. When I worked with him, I asked him questions about his mother, about their relationship and about losing her. His answers and his descriptions helped him process through his grief. Later, he told me that because of the pain his family felt, I was the only person he was talking to about his mother.

Whitt participated in sports and school activities, and helped his dad out at his business when time allowed. Like many other teenagers, staying busy helped him get through difficult times. To my surprise, one Friday morning at school Whitt, visibly shaken, came rushing into my office and sat down. He immediately started talking about an incident in P.E. that had just happened. I had never seen him this upset. As I was trying to understand what he was telling me, he looked up, looked me straight in the eyes, and said, "We never did go to the cemetery!"

I was taken back by the sudden switch in vocal tone and subject. "No, we never did," I said. Whitt asked, "Could we go now?" I replied, "But Whitt, look outside! It is cold, and it is raining a fine mist." He said, "It fits the mood." At this point I knew that I was going to have to get permission from the principal and Whitt's dad to allow us to visit the cemetery. Fortunately, it was just before Whitt's scheduled lunch and fifth-period elective.

Nothing had prepared me for the memorable experience I was about to share with Whitt when we visited his mother's grave at the cemetery. I had never done this with a student before. After a silent prayer, we walked and talked. It was a beautiful time. I did not rush him, and after 45 minutes, it was time to go.

Whitt had been talking a great deal since he had come into my office, and he continued at the cemetery. For the first time I told Whitt about meeting his mother before she died. I had refrained telling him earlier about talking with his mother to help his healing. It was important that Whitt remember and describe his mother as seen through his own eyes and experience. She had come to my office with her concern about Whitt regarding her illness. He was surprised I had visited with his mother, but not surprised at her concern for him.

When Whitt and I returned to school, the principal expected us to be depressed. Instead, I could not explain it, but we felt wonderful! When I arrived home after school, I was not my usual "end-of-the-week" tired. I told my husband I thought it strange that I had renewed energy and felt great. He assured me that the feeling resulted from a successful day that obviously helped Whitt. This day became the beginning of the last stage of recovery for Whitt.

ORGANIZING A GROUP

More students in our district were effected by grief that year. A high school student, Geoff, lost his mother in a car accident. I knew him because he had been in my seventh-grade honors English class.

Geoff worked for the local newspaper, and he wrote a touching article about losing his mother. When I read his article, I could tell he was in a great deal of pain. I immediately thought it would be a good idea to organize a high school grief group and combine it with a grief group from the middle school. First, I talked with Anna, and she encouraged me to contact Geoff. He was initially surprised, then, he decided he liked the idea. The two high school students talked with other students who had lost immediate family members. Tyler, a middle school student, and Megan, his sister in high school, wanted to join some type of group because their dad had been killed in a car accident.

At the first meeting, there were eight people in attendance. Geoff, Megan, Jason, and Anna were there from the high school. From the middle school, there were Whitt and Tyler. The high school counselor, Ann Middleton, and I facilitated the session. I was surprised that each person was so willing to take a risk and share. They did a great deal of talking.

The first four sessions went well, then scheduling and communication problems surfaced. The high school students had to go to jobs after school or they were in athletics. There was too large of an age difference within the group. The junior high students appeared to take conversations less seriously, perhaps to cover their true feelings, which aggravated the older group members. Transportation was also a problem, but meeting during the day was impossible because the two schools' schedules were incompatible.

One of the positive outcomes of the grief group was the fact all of the teenagers were writing as a means to process through some of their pain. Everyone, except Whitt, previously had used some form of writing to deal with his or her grief. These students were encouraged to continue writing, and eventually someone in the group suggested combining their work to benefit other grieving teenagers. The project developed quickly. When it became impossible to meet as a group, I met with each teenager individually and suggested continuing the writing project.

3

A Student's Untimely Death

A year later our community was confronted with a tragic death. Phillip, an eighth-grade student with three brothers, was killed in a car accident on a Saturday afternoon. Two other teenage boys in the car were injured, but survived.

The principal called me at home with the bad news. He planned to ask the agency that provides counseling for our district employees to be available at school Monday to visit with the students. When I hung up the phone, I received more calls. Teachers were being contacted by upset teenagers, and they were concerned. The teachers wanted a counselor to visit with their first-period classes Monday morning and address any problems that might occur because of Phillip's death.

Phillip was a well-liked, handsome kid. I was upset by his death, and I knew the news would have a rippling affect on the students. My greatest fear was that a distraught teenager might act out his grief for Phillip's death by committing suicide. I knew if this happened, other students might copy the behavior. Therefore, all decisions regarding the upset teenagers at school had to be evaluated from all angles.

There was no time to waste. I was concerned the agency counselors might be delayed getting to our school, and I knew the students would need our attention first thing Monday morning. I immediately called the elementary, primary, and two high school counselors. We decided to meet with the middle school teachers one half hour before classes to address their concerns. After the first bell, the counselors would divide the classes and discuss Phillip's death in each class for 15 minutes or longer if needed.

Our counselors arrived at the middle school early Monday morning. When I saw the principal, he told me the counseling agency was not coming. Their counseling was limited to district employees and their families. I was thankful our schools had developed a "disaster plan" for Phillip's death and this difficult situation could be dealt with quickly.

On their way to the library to speak to the middle school teachers, the counselors met three high school students. They appeared to be in shock as they walked down the hall with their arms around each other. They had been Phillip's friends. I do not think they knew what they were doing or where they were going. The high school is one block from the middle school and more high school students began entering the middle school. A counselor led the high school students back to their building where she visited with them.

Each time I spoke to a classroom, the students were quiet and did not react for about five minutes. Then, a few would cry, but most just sat there, finding Phillip's death hard to believe. Most of the time, teenagers think they are immortal. When a good friend dies, they must face the realities of life.

Phillip's Friends Meet As A Group

As I walked to my office, the computer instructor asked me to come to her classroom. She brought a group of students there after she found them huddled together crying in the hall. They had left their classes because they were too upset to stay.

There were twelve to fifteen boys and girls. Two boys were wearing large professional football-type jackets with the hoods pulled so far down that most of their faces were concealed. One boy had an arm around a crying girl who was leaning into his shoulder. Most of them were sitting there crying. A girl started pounding the table and repeated several times, "It's not fair! He was only fifteen! It's not fair!"

Someone answered, "No, it's not fair, but that's the way death sometimes happens, when we expect it the least." They talked about their anger for twenty minutes. When I felt the time was right, I had them move their chairs to form a circle where everyone could be seen and heard. Most of them wanted to describe how they reacted when they learned of Phillip's death. They listened to each other with care and respect. Everyone took his or her time, no one was rushed.

Then, the sharing centered around memories of Phillip. I was fascinated at how they cried at particular memories and laughed at others. The mood was intense, but they appeared to be thriving on the opportunity to express themselves and give support to others. At one point, they became very quiet, bowed their heads, and a boy said a prayer. I was touched to know that in a tragic situation such as this, they found comfort in prayer. Most people in this community attend Protestant churchs, so the traditions and beliefs center around the Bible and prayer.

After an hour, an eighth-grade girl gave me a poem she had written the night before for Phillip. For many people, writing about how they feel can be easier than trying to verbalize feelings, or it can act as a script for expressing how a person feels.

We Love You

The life that was taken cannot be replaced,
The tear stains will forever be on my face.
One life was taken and we can never forget
The terror of that fatal crash.
I cannot believe you're really gone,
Your life was no longer than the dawn.

When you die you look the same
Just as the day when your time came.
We will miss your beautiful eyes and
       handsome face,
Caring touch and well dressed taste.
We hope you knew that we all loved you.
We will always love and miss you too.

by Misty Welch

After I read the poem aloud, someone mentioned his concern for Phillip's mother. A sympathy card that one of the kids brought was passed around to get everyone's signature, but they wanted to write her messages too.

Making Phillip's Locker A Memorial

They spent another hour writing personal messages to Phillip's mother. Suddenly, a boy stood up and said he was going to put a lock on Phillip's locker. I suggested they put items in the locker that reminded them of Phillip, like Misty's poem. They immediately decided to include a Seven-Up, his favorite drink, and Cheetos, his favorite snack. They also chose a comb and a can of hair spray because Phillip always wanted to look good. Two or three boys left to get these items. In about five minutes, two more students left the room.

A few minutes later, the vice-principal entered shaking his head and smiling. He said the students did not want

Phillip's books in his locker, but did request the detention slip he received Friday so it could be placed in his locker. Soon the students returned with the articles. I asked if they wanted to have a short ceremony when they put the items in Phillip's locker. They thought it was a great idea, but they wanted all the eighth-grade students there. When they sought the principal's permission, he told them the ceremony was a good idea, but only for the small group who had planned it.

They were disappointed other students could not be included. Quietly, students started leaving and returning with a friend, or two, or three. Remembering Phillip in such a way was important to them and their friends. Our group of 15 grew to 40 or more.

In a few minutes, everyone went to Phillip's locker. Because there was a large number of students present, the students sat in front of Phillip's locker. Phillip's friends had planned the ceremony. They knew what they wanted to say and what they wanted to do. The first boy read a Bible scripture. The second boy described the significance of each item as he placed it in Phillip's locker. The third boy said a prayer. After the prayer, I looked to see teachers who had come into the hall. They too were affected by the tragedy and by the pain their students were feeling.

The principal spoke briefly about Phillip. He said that the lock would remain in place until the end of the school year when the items in the locker would be given to Phillip's mother. There was something about the click of the lock when it snapped shut that sounded and felt like a thud. In a way, that click signified the end. Students and teachers were crying and no one moved. After what seemed like an eternity, the bell rang and students started filling the halls. We were at the end of one hall, near an outside door. Teachers helped me move the emotionally upset students outside. The fresh air and sunshine felt good.

I realized I needed to "ground" or help these students recognize the importance of their tasks at hand before their afternoon classes. I felt the morning had been necessary and helpful, but now it was time to get them to concentrate on school. I took them back to the computer classroom where I told them we had one hour before lunch and I wanted them to attend their afternoon classes. I encouraged them to tell something funny that Phillip had done or said. If they chose not to participate, when it was their turn, they could say, "pass." No one passed. What they accomplished was not easy, and I must confess, some of their comments may have been considered "R-rated," but these kids laughed and laughed. They needed to laugh. When the lunch bell rang, they were ready and all of these students made it through their afternoon classes.

The locker was a memorial to Phillip and provided something concrete for kids to see and touch. They taped poems, notes, and flowers to his locker. The teachers respected the students' privacy when they saw them at his locker. Occasionally, a new note or poem would appear, and they remained there until summer break.

Friends Learn to Cope

Two days after the memorial service, eight students who were struggling with their emotions and having trouble concentrating, spent the morning in my office. Each one found support and love from the others. They expressed themselves freely, and no one felt shame when he cried. Amazingly, they were prepared to attend classes the rest of the day.

The next day, the same students were able to return to class after a short period of time. Each day was a struggle, but allowing students time at school to share and process their hurt and other feelings allowed them to move forward. If their feelings had been ignored or their needs not met, or if they had been rushed, their reactions could have been disastrous.

Adults need to be sensitive and realize that a teenager's death affects an entire community. There are many resources in the community (school counselors, psychologists, trained religious counselors, and hospice counselors) who are prepared to address problem areas families face during grief.

Phillip's close friend, Chad, returned to school the third day, and promptly visited me. He had some thought-provoking questions he obviously had spent a great deal of time considering. They all related to life after death. Chad asked, "If I live to be an old man before I die, and Phillip was 15 when he died, will we recognize each other in heaven? Will our age difference matter?"

Chad was seeking answers, and I knew that getting in touch with his feelings at this point was not his primary issue. I tried to be as honest as possible with him. I told him, "I feel strongly there is an essence about "heavenly beings" that will help us identify those we loved on earth but your preacher is better qualified to discuss this kind of topic." After listening intently, Chad looked up at me, smiled, and said, "Thank you."

Phillip's funeral was difficult, but his friends and teachers seemed to feel better the next week. Each week brought us closer to the school year's end. Each week I thanked God that our community experienced no more tragedies.

Phillip's Brother Reaches Out

The last week of school, a young mother who had recently lost her baby to "sudden infant death syndrome" came to school holding two small pieces of paper. The paper had been wrapped in plastic and carefully placed at the cemetery where the mother could find it. She wanted to meet the author, who turned out to be Phillip's brother, David. From the emotional support expressed in this letter and poem, grew a friendship based on mutual loss and understanding. Their friendship continues today.

Dear Whoever reads this,

I am deeply sorry for your loss and wish I could do more than a letter and poem. My brother died in March from a car accident and I know how it feels to lose someone you love. He was 15. His name is Phillip. I hope this poem gives you comfort. I know you don't know me, but I'm just concerned. My brother's grave is close to your son's. I'm pretty sure your son wouldn't want you to be sad, when he's in heaven having fun. He was probably a very smart and kind boy that will always be remembered. My teacher was talking to me and she said something that really made sense. She said, "We should cry when someone is born and rejoice when they die." I am in the 6th grade at Lake Dallas Middle School. I hope you get through the hard time, and remember you're in my prayers. If you need to talk, call me.

Love, David

Following is the poem David left for the baby's family at the cemetery.

For Comfort

How would it feel to lose a child?
Hope I'll never know.
The grief must be so very intense.
The tears would surely flow.

We want our loved ones here with us
So their lives we can share.
Not to be able to hold your child close
Must be almost too much to bear.

But then think of all the happiness
He must surely feel.
He will be with his Heavenly Father
And at His feet he'll kneel.

Your grief isn't for your son at all
Because in a better place he'll be.
The grief is for the loneliness you feel,
But you must set him free.

He has another mission to serve.
It was our Heavenly Father's plan.
He went to prepare a place for you
In a not so distant land.

His memory will always be with you
And soon the pain will ease.
The beautiful memories will come to the fore
And then there will be peace.

Families are forever, my friend,
And one day at Heaven's door
When your mortal life is over
You'll be with your son once more.

by Ann Mitchell   Springdale, Arkansas

4

Not Dealing With Grief

by Geoff Flowers

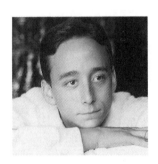

Geoff (pronounced "Jeff") Flowers was leader of the group project. He also kept extremely busy with school activities and his job at the local newspaper. During this time, he was recognized as an outstanding sports journalist and received an award. It took a long time, but he finally accepted and dealt with his mother's death.

The relationship between a parent and a child is very special. It is the first relationship for the child to base other relationships upon. The relationship between my mother and me was near perfect and awesome.

My name is Geoff Flowers. I was an eighteen-year-old senior at Lake Dallas High when I wrote this. My mother, Kathryn, was abruptly taken out of my life in the summer of 1993, after my junior year. I wish I could say it was just destiny that took her, but she died because somebody else was plain stupid.

On July 11 of 1993, my mother was riding in her boyfriend's truck on a small Oklahoma road. At about noon, they spotted her boyfriend's best friend in his one-ton truck coming down the opposite side of the same road. As a game, the two 36-year-old men liked to play "chicken." However this time, when one swerved, the other accidentally swerved the same way and they collided head on. Nobody was wearing a seat belt and both men had been drinking.

My mother and her boyfriend were knocked unconscious on impact and died a few minutes later. The best friend had his nine-year-old son in the truck with him. Both were critically injured and were unconscious at the scene.

The best friend was later indicted on charges of involuntary manslaughter. He received a few years probation and maybe his license was suspended. Whatever it was, it was too light.

My mother was the most caring person I ever had the pleasure of knowing. She was nice to everybody, but she had her moments. The only reason she was still with her boyfriend was because she cared about him too much.

My mom's boyfriend was a great guy. He was extremely nice, but he was addicted to pain killers and was an alcoholic. He told my mother if he died he would be buried under a small oak tree by his house. My mom asked him if she had never met him where would he be. He said six feet under the oak tree. That's why she stayed with him.

My mother raised me to the best of her ability. I can't tell you how much I loved my mother. I really didn't show it all the time, but I will never love anybody that much again. My future wife may get as much love, but it will be a different love.

My mother was the most influential person in my life. She taught me manners that few men still have. I open doors for ladies. I offer to pay for meals also. Whenever I see a girl cry, it makes me want to go over and see if I can cheer her up or help her out.

The most important thing my mother taught me was how to treat other people. I try to treat people with utmost respect, if they deserve it. Only a handful of people I have come across don't deserve respect because they treat others badly.

My mother loved the outdoors. She loved plants and on the weekend she worked in the yard trimming, fertilizing, or whatever needed to be done. It was a passion for her. At first, I really didn't care for it. After awhile I started to enjoy it. It kind of became a bonding time.

You can't really say I was a "Momma's boy." I have always been independent, but in a way I was dependent on her. I had to have her courage, nurturing, love, joy, and most importantly, I had to make her proud. Without it, I was half a person.

About the time my mom was killed on that small Oklahoma road, I was at a journalism camp in Addison, Texas and around 12:30 a.m., there was a knock at the door.

I got up and my advisor told me to get dressed and get in his room. I thought I was just switching rooms but that wasn't the case.

He came back and told me to get completely packed and dressed. A wave of fear engulfed me. "What was going on?" I kept asking myself. He came back in and said, "I hate to see this happen to a good kid like you." Then I asked, "Am I in trouble?" He said I wasn't, but I was partly right.

I looked up and saw my real dad in the door. He came right over to me and sat down. "Geoff, your mom is dead," he said. I wish he had put it a better way, but it got the point across.

I fell out of my chair and knelt on the floor. I cried, yelled and screamed, but worst of all, I felt completely alone. My real father picked me up and got me together. As I was leaving, my advisor told me something I will never forget: "Vaya con Dios" which is Spanish for "Go with God."

I had met my real dad only a year before my mom died. He was a nice guy, but he didn't fill the reason I looked him up and called him, which was to have a father.

Up until the time my mother died, my real dad and I had an off and on relationship. I had to do all the talking. I always had to call him. It got bothersome because he never called me.

About a year before my mom died, she and my step-dad separated. She and I moved closer to the school. She left him mostly because of me. I told her to do it because she wasn't happy. I wish I hadn't. My step-dad was a great guy, but he just didn't spend enough time with me. Plus, he and my mother were having problems. She cried all the time so, I hated him for it. That's when I decided to find out who my real dad was.

After my mom died, I had a few choices on where to live. I could live with my real dad, my step-dad or my grandmother. I chose the best choice, my step-dad. He really was my father. The court said he was too when he adopted me in December of 1993.

Now our relationship is very close. I don't see him every day, but at least once a week we sit down and have a good talk. We really haven't talked about my mother much, but we both know and agree on one thing: we really miss her.

By the time I got home the night of the accident, my older sister was there. I walked in and we just hugged each other and cried. About twenty minutes later my grandfather walked in. We all just hugged each other and cried. My youth minister and my boss came over to see if I was all right. My step-dad called, and my sister and I talked to him.

We all sat around until about 4:00 in the morning. My dad and youth minister left and the rest of us tried to get some sleep. That was absolutely the longest night of my life. I sat there in bed and cried for the last time. I haven't cried like that since.

I got about an hour of sleep that night. I woke up the next day in the hopes that mom was still alive, but I knew right away she wasn't. I felt so empty and I just wanted to cry. For some reason, I didn't.

Before my mother died, I didn't cry much. I liked to laugh a lot, but I really didn't show much emotion. It took a lot to make me mad. Now, I have an incredibly short fuse and anything can bring me down.

I used to have a high emotional tolerance, but now I can't take too much abuse. I tend to blow up at people a lot more. Don't get me wrong. I still love to laugh. It helps me relax and deal with myself. I love to make other people happy when I can't be. It helps to try to cheer me up.

Whenever I hear a sad song, I get depressed. I feel everything I felt that night all over again. It makes me feel so helpless.

The funeral was a rough time. Everybody was on edge and mad about how she died. A couple days before the funeral, I wanted to go see my mother, but my grandmother wouldn't let me. She said my mother's face was bruised and puffy from the wreck. I understood and all, but I really wanted to say good-bye one last time.

My step-dad and sister took my mother's death very hard. At the funeral, he just held her picture and cried. He kept carrying it around and showing it to everybody. My sister was a wreck. She took it real hard. She just wasn't herself. I can't explain it.

Everybody took the death as expected, except me. I took it very well, too well. I didn't let it ruin my schedule. I kept the family going and made sure that everything flowed well. I was even the last person to the funeral to make sure everybody was there.

I wish I had dealt with the death then instead of not dealing with it. It took a lot out of me. I lost my ability to push myself over the limits. I stopped caring about what I did. I was doing a mediocre job in everything I was doing. About March, it all caught up with me.

I fell into a deep depression. I didn't care about anything except my writing and the people I cared about. I just wanted to be by myself, so when I wasn't at school, I just did stuff by myself.

A few months before all this started, Janet Tyson approached me about forming the grief group. She decided it was time to form one after she read a story in the newspaper I wrote about my experiences. The group met for the first time with six people and it was pretty successful.

At first, nobody would talk, but after awhile somebody broke the barrier and said something. After that, we all opened up and started to talk. We all learned a lot, but we also heard a lot of stuff that we already knew. It wasn't until we started on the book that we learned the most about ourselves.

I loved writing in the book. It was an escape for me. Whatever I was writing, it made me feel better. I worked at a small newspaper in Lake Dallas. I covered high school sports for them. I also worked on the school newspaper. I wrote a lot for them also. Somehow, whenever I was writing it made me feel better. To this day I still don't know how or why.

After I made it through my own version of March Madness, I found a job at a movie theater. I loved it. It was the perfect job for me. I love to see movies, so it was the ideal job since I got free movies. I became one of their most important employees. I often worked fifty hours a week while I finished my junior year. Now that I look back, I was only working to stay busy so I didn't have to deal with my problems.

The job at the theater helped me a lot. I met a lot of people who are now close friends. I do things with them more than with the people at school.

After I started my senior year, I was working two jobs---the newspaper and the theater---going to school, and working on the yearbook staff. It turned out I was working seven days a week at least sixty hours. I was so busy that I didn't have time to do much of anything except work.

After football season ended, I quit the newspaper job and worked just for the theater. I still worked sixty hours a week, but I had Mondays off. It was a routine I had fallen into, and one I was afraid of getting out of. March Madness started all over again except it was November.

All I wanted to do was die. I hated life at that point. The way I was looking at it nothing in my life was going right. A lot of my friends were pretty worried about me. I wasn't the same person. I didn't care about myself. I would have given my life up in a heartbeat to save another person but I had planned my own suicide several different ways. The only thing that kept me from doing it was I the pain I knew it would cause. I only wanted to cause myself pain.

I started to see a counselor at the high school. She helped me turn my life around by teaching me new strategies. It took five months of long conversations before school, during lunch, or whenever we could go talk.

I learned a lot about me. I am a fairly complex person. I am pretty stubborn about my thinking. I think one way, and it takes a miracle to change it. I learned how to open myself. I never did it before because I didn't want to get hurt again. I learned that I had to be my own person, not somebody else's. Work, school, and the yearbook were running my life, not me. I had to change that.

I cut back my hours at work. I did a lot more things with my friends which I couldn't do before. I spent some time by myself to get my life back on track. That was a chore in itself. It is real hard to get by yourself, especially when there are only 24 hours in a day.

I have now finished high school and graduated. I really didn't think I would live to see the day when I would receive my diploma. When I finally got the diploma, I broke down and cried. I had to shake hands and hug all the teachers. My family and extended family saw me, and they all started to cry.

I have signed with the United States Navy and will be starting on August 9th. It will be a great experience for me and I can't wait to go. The only problem is that I will have to leave all my friends and my family for six years. Another problem is that I have a girlfriend and I have to leave her too.

Words of Encouragement:

Take time and deal with the death instead of not dealing with it.

5

Long Illness Doesn't Make Loss Easier

by Whitt Keyes

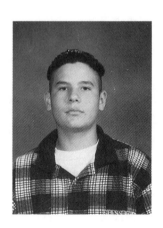

Whitt Keyes, like his Native American ancestors, is a proud individual who keeps thoughts and feelings to himself. He worked several months on his project and once he developed trust, he wrote and talked at length. His progress was most evident. Now, he is in high school in another district doing an outstanding job in athletics. He frequently calls or comes by our school to see everyone.

The worst day of my life was when I found out that my mom had died. We always had a good relationship because we spent a lot of time together. Our favorite activity was shopping at the mall. Sometimes we stayed at one store for hours. It was fun most of the time except when my feet would get tired. As a result of shopping all of the time, my mom dressed nice. She also made me dress nice, and if she didn't like it, she wouldn't let me wear it. Driving to the mall was fun too because we talked about my life, and sometimes, her's.

My mom thought our family was the most important thing in her life. She spent a lot of time with her family. I can remember playing soccer. She used to cheer for me all of the time. If she saw some grown-up yelling at me, she would jump on them and make them stop. She would encourage me to go after what I wanted. Most of the time I accomplished it.

My mom loved listening to country music. Although I didn't like country music, I still listened to it because of her. She was also very talented. She sewed for hours making clothes for herself and my little sister. She loved to sew. A lot of people really liked my mom. Of course, running a day care for children, she had to be liked.

My name is Whitt. I am in the seventh grade. My mom played a big part in my life. She encouraged something very important to me: my braided tail. It's about two feet long on the back of my head. It's important to me because I've been growing it since kindergarten. For eight years, I've had it. I have a braided tail because I am Native American from my dad's side. Out of the five civilized tribes, I belong to the Choctaw tribe which originated from Mississippi.

October 20, 1992, was when my mom died. My sister was three years old. It was rough....It is still rough.

I was with Mother at the doctor's office when she found out about the lump in her breast. It was at the end of my fourth-grade year. The next week, the doctor operated.

That morning we got up at 4 am to be at the hospital for a 6 am operation. I thought it was no big deal and that my mom would be out soon. I sat in the waiting room and watched t.v. It turned out that she was in the operating room eight hours.

The doctor talked to Dad, Grandmother, and Grandfather after lunch. Dad took me outside the hospital and told me that the problem was not an infection, but was cancer. I knew it was serious because everyone was crying. I think Mom was told first.

Mom came home from the hospital early the next morning. Things resumed like they had been....for a while. Then, Mother started chemotherapy therapy. Her hair started falling out and that hurt me. I don't like to remember her like that.

Fifteen months later, she began to sleep more and get sick, this meant her condition was getting worse. Two days before she died, she went to the hospital while I was still in school. When I visited with her in the hospital, she was sitting up in a chair. I had mixed feelings about her using a breathing machine to help keep her alive because I didn't want to see her suffer.

When she was in the hospital, I kept thinking she would be home soon until the last day. I went home from the hospital at 6 p.m., but Dad stayed. They told me Mom wouldn't live through the night.

The next day at school, they called me out of third period. Dad was at school. I asked him if we were going to see Mom and he said, "She died."

On Wednesday we went to her service. Friends and relatives were there. Mrs. White, my school teacher, and Scott, my friend, were there. People brought food and visited at home. It helped me to get out of the house and throw the football with my cousins.

The past two years have been hard, but now times have gotten easier. Keeping busy has helped me. I've been playing sports like baseball, football, and basketball. I've worked hard to be good in all of them. I am on the "A--B" honor roll and I am in the excel class for math. My sister, Jeanaka, who is five, is doing fine in cheerleading, gymnastics, and dancing. My dad played in a national tournament this year in Dallas for fast pitch softball. My dad and I are close. He coached my baseball team this past summer and now we are planning a trip to Mexico.

After high school, I plan to go to college at Michigan or Miami and play sports. Hopefully, I'll continue my career in the pros.

Words of Encouragement:

Don't think about the death all of the time. There are times you have to be busy, or lose your mind.

6

Remembering & Healing

by Megan Ray

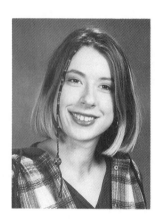

Megan Ray is a dramatic, bubbly, outgoing girl, who uses a dramatic style to express herself. Her writing reveals the importance of her family. When the group was meeting, she discovered she needed a great deal of time to reflect and process what she had written. Megan graduated from high school and plans to go to college this fall.

Memories are carried on a warm summer's breeze
to remind me of things past.
I need them to survive and thrive.
This is my story.

I will never forget the day I saw my father in his coffin. He looked so unnatural, so cold, and yet so peaceful. It hurt a lot to see him that way. And now looking back, I would like to mend the feelings that went sour between us. No one is as close as my father was to me.

I think I treasure my family's love more than anything. As a result of my father's death, I hold my family near and dear to my heart. It would be so hard to lose another family member. Most people would laugh in my face to see the way I treasure them. I don't treat them like royalty, just respectfully. When you have a big loss, it opens your eyes to the world around you and you see what you have left. And, you think, "Oh my God, is this all?"

My name is Megan. I was born on January 6, 1978 in Colorado. I can remember the rope swing my mother put up in our living room. I used to pretend that I was a princess and that the swing was my "get away" into the great gray forest. Another thing I remember was drying my hair in the heat vents of that same house. One day I saw Mom drying her hair, so I guess I decided to be a "copy cat."

I also remember the Fourth of July our family watched fireworks from our roof! It was great. I loved Colorado so much. Colorado has ice blue skies and majestic mountains. The party ended when we moved to Texas. Mom said I practiced my Texas twang all the way down here. I would give anything in the world to move back. My grandma lives in Colorado, along with my aunt and my cousin.

There are many more memories. I remember when my brother was born. I wanted to name him, but none of my names suited my parents. Some of the strange names included Peter Rabbit, Juniper Tree, and Brier Fox. Now, my brother is the person I most admire. He alone is a single guiding light in the night....a special star in the sky....the real McCoy. He doesn't know what I think of him and I would like to keep it that way.

Most people take memories for granted. I have very special memories of my father, like our wrestling matches, going to Six Flags, Wet and Wild, movies, and dancing. My dad was a great guy.

My dad died about 4:00 a.m. on Thursday, October 3, 1991. My parents had just separated. So, Mom, Tyler, and I moved in with my Texas grandma.

That morning, I woke up, I don't know why, I just did. It was about 5:00 am and about five minutes later, the phone rang. I thought that it was Mom (who worked nights), but it was some guy who wanted to speak to Mom. I finally got him to talk to me. I was the first to find out about my father's death. From the other side of my house, my grandma heard me blurting out questions to the man on the phone. My grandma came in and asked me what was wrong. When I told her what had happened, she got on the phone and got the details. Twenty to 30 minutes later, Mom called to make sure we got up for school. When she found out that Dad had been in an accident, she made a 30 minute drive in ten minutes.

Dad fell asleep while driving and was hit head-on by a gravel truck. He was killed instantly. There were no last words, no scream, nothing. The truck driver got out with just a few scratches. Both vehicles were towed away. Because my father was killed on a highway where lots of accidents occur, he became just another statistic.

Thinking back, I don't remember how I felt after the phone call because everything was in confusion. It's just a blur. I will remember the hurt I had later, and there will always be a twinge of sadness in the future when my children ask about their grandfather.

Petals of a Flower

Petals are soft.
They remind me of my father's gentle touch.
I loved him dearly.
Now that he's gone,
I wish I could have more time to spend
with feelings to mend.
The scents I smell, remind me
of him.

page 45

Since I started our grief support group, a lot has gone on in my life. I am a junior in high school and my main interest is passing classes at school so I can graduate. One of my favorite activities is playing in the band. Several of us refer to the group of kids in the band as "The Mud Puddles." It's been over four years since my father died. In the beginning, I was packing my suitcase every other weekend to go visit him, and now I don't even remember his death date until days afterwards. After awhile all of the bad memories go away and all you can remember are the good memories.

I am going to work hard to become a marine biologist. I'll go to college and take the required courses. Who knows, one of these days I might help save the dolphins or discover a rare sea creature. It would be good to make a contribution to mankind.

Words of Encouragement:
Take one day at a time and don't be ashamed to cry.

7

Dealing With Grief
Through Letters

by Tyler Ray

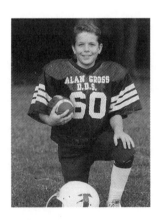

Tyler Ray, the youngest member of the original grief group, quickly completed his section of the project. He has the unique ability to state exactly how he feels, and as you will see, used a unique method to do so. In all areas of his life, he continues to develop and experience success.

My name is Tyler, and Megan is my sister. I was born in Colorado on July 29, 1982. Soon after I was born, my family moved to Texas. The first memory I ever had was when I was four years old. I had the best Christmas I can ever remember. In those days my sister and I usually got everything we wanted for Christmas. I got electronic toys and my sister got Barbies and girl stuff like that. Now days, we are low on money and don't have much.

The first birthday I remember was when I was five. I had a birthday party at McDonald's and invited all of my first grade friends. Each person had two hamburgers and a large order of French fries. Everyone had fun looking through the styrofoam hamburger boxes for little plastic rings. We had to push a button to get the merry-go-round to spin and play music. Everyone had a great time.

When Megan and I were kids, we would climb up on a closet shelf and tell ghost stories. Now, my sister is 15 years old and she won't do things like that anymore. She always goes out with her friends and never spends time with me. Sometimes I don't know what to feel...lonely, happy, scared, frustrated, mad, sad, left out, or even abandoned.

When I was younger, I remember how shy of pictures my dad was, and how he gave a fake smile. He wore very strong glasses because his vision was bad. Sometimes my dad would take my sister and me bowling or to the movies. He influenced me to be a guitarist because he was the lead singer with a rock group in Colorado. Dad would always joke with us when Megan and I were in the car. We would hit him in the arm. At home we would wrestle Dad to the ground and "play" beat him up.

Every summer we would go with Dad to Oklahoma to a camping place called Chickasha National Park. At the park they have nature hikes and ice cold springs. I remember a ten foot waterfall, maybe taller, with foot holes in the rock wall just large enough for my feet. When I reached the top of the falls, I would dive like a "dare devil." When we got tired of the water falls, we would go further down on the nature trails. My favorite place in the park was where we camped near a two foot water fall with about 30 feet of playing room. Behind the shallow waterfall were cliffs that were good for jumping into the water. The park rangers finally posted a sign that said it would be a fifty dollar fine if caught jumping from the cliffs. That really spoiled my fun.

When my mom and dad separated two months before his death, my dad moved out of our house. He did not have much money so he ate Hamburger Helper, tuna fish, and bologna sandwiches. My sister and I knew our diet would consist of one of these choices when we visited him, but it didn't matter because I really loved my dad.

Then one morning I slept late on a school day. When I finally woke up, I went into my mom's room. She had just come in from work and had an unusual look on her face. She motioned for me to come to her. I could see she was trembling. I asked my mother what was wrong. She said, "Tyler, your father is dead." I fell to the ground, bursting with tears. My mother said it was okay and I would get over it. I said, "Not this! I will never get over this." She told me that I did not have to go to school, but I decided that it was best for me to go.

We went to the funeral home on a Friday evening. My mom said that I should not go, but I said, "No, I am going. It is the last chance I will get to see him." When we got to the funeral home, I didn't believe he was really there. Once I got through the doors where the coffin was, I saw him. That's when I believed for the first time he was dead.

Today I am concentrating on school and passing. Band is my favorite extracurricular activity. Whenever I am not doing homework, I usually go outside and play football. Whenever it gets warmer in the season, we play baseball and tennis. I also have a hobby building small models and working on electrical fans. I usually get the parts from junk yards.

In the future I want to go to high school and get a scholarship for football, golf, or tennis. When I go to college, I want to go to the University of Southern Carolina, Duke, or Notre Dame. It would be great if I could be in the NFL or the Air Force.

Now, when I'm in school, the feeling I have is normal and natural. I am not saying that whenever someone makes fun of my dad or brings him up, I don't get defensive. I am saying that I don't break out and cry in class.

One thing I did to help me after my dad's death was write notes to my dad and let him know what was on my mind. I am going to burn the letters so the smoke can carry my messages to him. Here are samples of some of my letters:

October 4

Dear Dad,

How is life in paradise? Our cat had two litters of kittens. Keep a record of this because I will be writing many more letters and burning them so you can read them.

Tomorrow is our field trip at school. We are going to see the Aladdin play. I have made a new friend. His name is David.

Dad, do me a favor. Ask God (if you ever see him) why he chose October 3, 1991, for you to die. Ask him why he didn't let you live until you were old and ready to die. I sure do miss you. I will never forget that miserable day when Mom told me you were dead. If I had believed it that day, I would have cried more.

Love you very much,

Tyler

P.S. I love you.

October 18

Dear Dad,

If you don't already know, in our counseling group, my sister and I are writing a book about you. I really have missed you over the years that you have been dead.

Megan has gone nuts. She dyed her hair red and dresses weird to go with it. Really stupid, isn't it? If I get a recent picture of her, I will send it to you.

Love you very much,
Tyler

P.S. Love you, miss you

November 15

Dear Dad,

Today, David and I got into a fight. I can't find my final draft that we had to write today. Everything is going to the birds this year. I can hardly pass science. Remember when you were alive and I went to Sanger schools? I used to make A's and B's all year. I don't know what has happened. Now, I am making C's, D's, and E's, and sometimes F's.

Love you,
Tyler

February 16

Dear Dad,

Yesterday I made a new record in golf. I hit the ball 136 ft. I also started a new book called *The Time Machine*. It is so good, I can hardly put it down. My mom bought me two really great books yesterday.

Love you,
Tyler

March 3

Dear Dad,
      Today is a good day. I am very happy and hyper. I made the school's honor roll. I hope I don't get into any trouble because I am so hyper. The table I sit at is so crowded I can't write without touching someone.
      Love you,
      Tyler

Words of Encouragement:

      My advice to a boy my age who has had a father die is, work hard to let him go. If you hang on, you will start to do poorly in school. I hung on to my dad so much I thought I saw him drive by the school in the truck.

8

Didn't Get to Say Good-bye

by Jason Hite

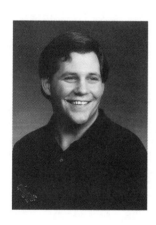

Jason Hite was the oldest student in our grief group. He tried to be independent both emotionally and financially by working very hard at two jobs after school and on weekends. He was active in group meetings and often took the lead in expressing himself. He has had a difficult time coping with guilt related to his mother's death. He has a positive attitude and continues to work hard in order to save money for college.

"Son, son, come on. I want you to come with us." I heard those words as I slowly opened my eyes.

"Mom, it's five a.m. I just went to bed! I'll see you when you get back. Shoot, Mom, you'll only be gone for three weeks," I said.

"I know, but I want you to come with your father and me," my mother prodded.

I answered her sharply, "I'll call Uncle Johnnie later today, so...goodnight!"

Later that day, I talked with my mom. She was disappointed in me, but she did understand. My father and brother were leaving the next day to visit family in Ohio. I thought that it was cool to stay with my sister-in-law. She doesn't boss me around or tell me to do chores. I was sixteen and I thought I knew everything.

My father told me where the emergency money was stashed. He also told me that he was leaving early in the morning and, "If you get busted, stay there and pray I don't find out!"

Everything went according to schedule for about a week or two. Then, I didn't hear anything from my mother for about three days. So, my sister-in-law and I decided to call her.

"What's wrong?" I asked as I looked at my sister-in-law's distorted face. She dropped the phone and stared into space. I ran outside not knowing what to think. Tears were running down my face.

I knew that something was wrong, but was afraid to ask. I walked slowly inside the house. My sister-in-law told me that my mother had an accident. I thought of catching a plane to be with my mother.

Instead, we called family and friends to tell them what we knew. That night my father came home with my oldest brother. It was the first time any of us had seen our father cry aloud.

Then my father called the airport to get tickets to fly back to Mom. My brother and I talked, but yet, neither was paying attention to the other.

The next morning, my father, brother and I took a flight to see how bad Mom was. She was on life support and was never expected to get any better. She had zero brain activity.

Together we decided to unplug the machine. It was the hardest decision we've ever had to make. At 8:33 a.m. the doctor turned the machine off. The young 46-year-old woman would never see another sunrise.

That's when I realized that my mom was gone. I was all alone, nobody to help me. The last time I saw my mother, I was bitching at her for waking me up. This was something I will have to live with for the rest of my life.

She is gone. I am alone in the dark, just staring at the ceiling, not knowing what to do next. My alarm rings a high pitched scream. My father walks into the room and says, "It is time."

Slowly I reach to turn the alarm off. My father shakes his head and turns to walk out. I get up, take a shower, and then get dressed. As I walk through the hall, I hear, "I'm sorry," about a dozen times.

There is confusion running through my mind. Not knowing is the worst feeling a person can feel. The words, "She is gone," echo in my mind. I just can't understand how I could have been with her one night and not the next. The people around me say they understand, but do they just say it to make me feel better?

I went to the funeral home with my father to pick out a coffin. I didn't show how much I was hurting; I just smiled and said, "That is a nice one there."

I remember being in a daze. The funeral is two days away. I go to the mall from the funeral home. I have to grab a suit to wear. The images of her face cloud my mind. I find a nice gray suit to wear.

As I get out of the car at home, I notice there are more cars than when I left. I just shake my head and walk to the front door. I see people from my hometown. I tell them I am doing all right. Deep down inside I know I will never be the same.

I go to my room to try to sleep, knowing it will never happen. As I lie on my bed, I think about her. She did everything for me. Every time I had a problem, I went to her. Now, who will I go to? I fade back into reality.

At the funeral home, I look down for the first time. She looks so different, not like her at all. I try to hide the tears falling down my face. I fall to the floor, and just sit there, staring into space. I feel so alone. No one understands the pain I am going through. I get up, wipe off the tears and say, "Good-bye," for the last time.

We must learn to live with death and be thankful for every day we are here. Remember to tell the one you love, how much you truly care. You never know if you'll get that chance tomorrow. I wish every day that God would give me just five minutes to say, "Good-bye" to my mother. But I know I'll never get that chance.

Words of Encouragement:
Just take one day at a time. Everything will fall into place.

9

Unexpected Loss

by David Levine

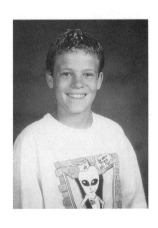

David Levine, brother of Phillip who was killed in a car accident, is in high school now. It gave him strength to attend support groups and help others in grief. From his experience, he contributes the following words of encouragement.

When I was ten years old, my mother told my brothers and me that my dad was moving out and they were getting a divorce. That was the worst time in my life. I hated my parents for not being together. I wouldn't talk to anyone and I was really depressed.

Six months later, my parents decided to try again and get back together. We moved to Arkansas where my dad had relocated for his job. Those were the best three months of my life. Then, my mom said we were moving back to Texas. I was more depressed than ever, but I hid my feelings inside. We moved back to into the trailer we had left in Texas.

After we moved back, my two older brothers made friends with a sixteen-year-old. He had a Chevy Blazer and my brothers loved to drive around with him. One afternoon, when I was in the sixth-grade, my brother Phillip was riding in the Blazer with two friends. They were going too fast while turning a wet corner and ran into a telephone pole. Phillip died on impact.

When I found out about the accident, I was in shock. I went to two different counselors to deal with my grief. My life has never been the same since the day my brother died. We did not discuss my brother's death at home. My mom was way more protective and wouldn't let me do anything unless she was there. She was afraid that the same thing would happen to me.

After a year, I was doing better. I helped start the grief support group with the school counselor and a few other kids who had family members pass away. Two years later, I am just like other kids my age. I like being with my friends and going places. I like going to parties and eating and sleeping. In the future, I plan to finish high school, go to college, and get a degree in teaching or business management.

Words of Encouragement:

Take one day at a time and live each day to its fullest. I think, personally, this statement is strong and if you live up to it, you will be too. Express your feelings. I believe it's good to express your feelings to a counselor or someone close who you trust. Every feeling you have is okay and normal. Don't let anyone tell you what you're feeling is wrong. It's "your" feeling.

I found that helping people through their grieving comforted me. Talking, listening, and sharing feelings with others in the counseling group at school helped me, and I believe it helped them, too. I also found that counseling groups offered in the community were fun and helpful.

10

Losing A Twin

by Kari Deakins

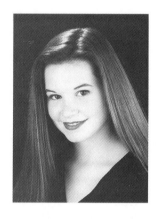

Few people understand the strong bond that is created at conception and lasts a life time for twins. Dr. Brandt, director of Twinless Twins Support Group International, introduced me to Kari Deakins. She vividly describes this bond that exists between twins in her story.

Hi! My name is Kari Deakins and I'd like to try and help you through this tough thing called grief. I'm still grieving myself, and trust me, it is something to be reckoned with.

I was born the first of fraternal twins, November 22, 1978, in Des Moines, Iowa. Can you believe that my mom didn't even know she was going to have twins until ten days before we were born?! Yep, "she" became "they," and we became Kari Elizabeth and Shari Anne.

When we were only six weeks old we moved to a tiny town in Oklahoma called Grove. My dad is a doctor and he had a small practice there. My two older brothers, Shari, and I had lots of fond memories of Grove, like dance class, church, my baby-sitters, lots of good friends, and of course, the daily fighting and bickering between my sister and me. Being fraternal twins, Shari and I were as different as night and day. We had an ongoing war, day in and day out, but hey, that's what sisters are for, right?

When we were five, my father joined the Navy and we moved from this tiny town to Pensacola and then Jacksonville, Florida. A near tragedy brought Shari and me closer for a while. Our mother was in a terrible car accident while our father was out to sea. She was hospitalized for what seemed like a year at least. We cried together hoping for our mom to recover quickly. Our older brothers were in college and high school and tried to look out for us. Fortunately, mother soon got better.

After our fifth-grade year, we had a big surprise! My dad was being stationed overseas and we were moving to Japan. For once Shari and I agreed on something, we didn't want to go! But, unfortunately, eleven-year-olds don't have a big say in those kinds of decisions. Our new home was in Yokosuka, Japan. WOW! What an experience!

At first Shari and I hated it, but we both grew to love it. We attended DODDS school on the base and made new friends. Shari and I had some classes together, but for the most part we had different friends and hobbies, but that changed as we grew older. We both shared a love for music, she continued to sing and I played in the band. We seemed to have more and more in common. We both made lots of friends and surprisingly had the same group of best friends. We were there for each other when we needed help and we stuck up for each other when we were in trouble. I think that's what's really important.

As we neared the end of eighth-grade, Shari was losing weight. For someone that had always been a little overweight, we were happy for her and her success. We all thought she was having great success with her exercising and healthful eating. In hindsight, we saw how anemic she looked and how often she was sick. Those should have been warning signs, but nothing seemed out of the ordinary.

By now we were quite settled in Japan and not ready to leave, but we moved back to Pensacola in July of 1993. Shari didn't feel well most of the time and she slept a lot. We really couldn't figure it out, but mostly attributed it to all the traveling that we'd been doing. While on vacation that summer in Columbia, Missouri, Shari got worse. Her right leg swelled to twice its normal size. She was taken to the hospital when the swelling didn't subside, and they found a large blood clot in her leg.

The doctors said that Shari had a Wilm's Tumor in her right kidney. I was horrified. I didn't know what to do. A few days later Shari was diagnosed with cancer, instead of having a Wilm's tumor. She had cancer of the kidneys, renal cell carcinoma. This cancer baffled everyone since renal cell carcinoma is usually only found in older people.

The doctors spent 12 hours in surgery to remove the cancer tumor. The tumor was HUGE, a little larger than a football. It weighed five pounds! There were never any warning signs. How could this have happened?!

Then came the waiting and recovery. Since Shari was in the hospital we couldn't go back to Pensacola to start school, so, I started high school in Missouri. I felt so lost. I was trying to absorb everything surrounding my sister's sudden illness. I had a really hard time at first, I wanted to curl up and just make it all go away!

When we left Japan, we lost our close knit community. Our entire support system was across an ocean from my sister and me. We kept in touch with our friends and they helped us to keep going. To help our family, our friends put together a fund raising dance. In Japan they started the Shari Deakins Scholarship Fund at our school.

Shari was in and out of the hospital, mostly undergoing chemotherapy and radiation. She was always worn out from constantly battling this illness. She grew thinner and thinner, apart from the constant swelling of parts of her body, usually in her lower half. She lost most of her hair and almost all of her body fat. Her mouth always had sores from the chemo and her breathing became very shallow and labored. It's sad that it took a life threatening illness to bring us closer. We talked all the time when she was awake, which became less often. Our arguing and our differences seemed to be resolved all of a sudden. I always carried the hope that she would get better, I never did believe them when they told me she would die.

In August of 1993, when she was diagnosed, the doctors told us Shari wouldn't make it to Thanksgiving, but she did. She lasted longer than they'd expected and continued to fight. We celebrated our 15th birthday in the hospital with a few friends. Then, the doctors didn't think she'd make it to Christmas, but she did. She made it past Valentine's, and almost to St. Patty's Day in March.

Shari's last months were really hard. She grew more emaciated above the waist and more swollen below. She was constantly in pain. It's hard to see someone so close to you die slowly and painfully. I never gave up the hope, I believed she would get better. But she never did, only worse. I guess I'm a pretty optimistic person anyway, but without optimism, my loss would have been much harder.

On Tuesday, March 15, 1994, at 8 p.m., Shari lost her battle with cancer. For the first time, my parents were away from her side at my chorus concert. Our pastor and his wife were staying with her at our house. They beeped my dad during my concert to tell him. When we got home she was already gone. Father Chris said Shari couldn't leave us while we were there, she had to wait for those she loved to be gone. She had said to him once that she was not afraid of dying, she was only afraid for those she would leave behind. My dad told me that at four that morning she awakened and he was by her side. Shari told him she loved him and then she drifted into a coma. That night she was gone forever.

I didn't believe it, I couldn't. It took a long time for it to sink in. I called all of our close friends and we cried together. It still seemed so unreal. It seemed as if she was just at the hospital again or something, it didn't feel so real yet. I just couldn't believe that she was gone for good. Her funeral was four days later.

Watching them put Shari in the ground was excruciating. A part of me went with her, and a part of her will always be in me. For a while I felt really numb, I couldn't feel the pain or the sorrow, nothing. Then, as everything started to sink in, I wanted to fall apart and make it all go away. It had finally hit me, Shari was never coming home, at least not to mine.

I knew that Shari was with me all the time after she passed away. That month I had a lot to do and she helped me every step of the way. I feel her always with me, especially when I sing.

It's been two years now since Shari died. WOW! Two years. It seems so long ago and yet it feels like yesterday. I still have a hard time believing she's gone forever. Not a day goes by that I don't think about her. My twin, my sister, sometimes even my friend, is gone, but she is still very much a part of my life.

My sixteenth birthday was hard. It was my first birthday without her, and it felt a little empty. Sometimes I think about how she didn't get to go to high school or to the dances like me. She didn't really get to date, or do everything I did. She wasn't here to order class rings or to go to the prom, and she won't be here for graduation. I can't imagine graduating without her. Healing is an ongoing, never ending process.

My mom pointed out this year that I "dealt" with my pain by not dealing with grief, which is not a good way to heal from this kind of loss. I stay so busy that I don't have any time to feel the hurt or pain that otherwise comes out. But, I believe that everything happens for a reason. It's God's will.

Please don't think that you are alone. Even if no one around you can understand your pain, others do. Without the support of my loving friends and family, I wouldn't be where I am today. But most of all I need God to help me understand and survive. I couldn't have handled Shari's death without my belief. I understand it's not God's "fault" that Shari's gone, I believe it was His plan all along. He needed her, and it was her time.

I've watched my parents and family suffer with me and we all help each other with our grief. Talking about everything with someone close to you helps more than you know. Bottling things up can only make it come out later and make things harder. Actually I'm pretty good at keeping my grief to myself, but I'm working on it. Writing is a great source of therapy.

Every once in a while I just break down and cry. I have good days more than bad days with my grief now, and it's easier than it used to be. Shari's room is still called that and many of her things still remain. My brothers are grown and we stay in close touch. Although physically gone, Shari lives in our hearts and always will.

Just remember that you're not alone and everyone needs help sometimes. It does get easier, it really does, and everyone grieves differently. Never let anyone tell you you've grieved enough or not enough. It takes everyone different periods of time to get "over" a great loss like that of a close friend or family member. Not that you ever get "over" it, but you do learn to live with it. You can't blame yourself or those around you, it's not your fault or theirs, it's just life. No one ever guaranteed that life would be fair.

Memory of Shari Anne Deakins

Today Shari's been gone a year,
As I remember I shed a tear.
We say a prayer and dry our eyes,
It feels to me, no time's passed by.
Tell me, has it been that long?
It seems so odd, it feels so wrong.

Though life goes on without her,
She is always here.
Her smile, her joy, her laughter
Her love are all still here.

My sister, yes, my friend, I pray,
Although we fought night and day.
If I said black, she said white,
And back and forth through all the night.

Different as we were
And hateful--so we thought,
I know that I have loved her,
And I think of her a lot.

I think of things she used to do,
With love and joy...and sadness too.
To run, to laugh, and just have fun,
She got along with most anyone.

She also loved to sing and act,
She was quite good as a matter of fact.
All to shortly she was here,
Fifteen years...just fifteen years!

by Kari Deakins, March 15, 1995

Words of Encouragement:

Express your emotions and feelings and get it all out. Keeping a journal is a good idea or writing poetry. Honest, it helps, and this way, you don't have to show it to anyone if you don't want to. It can be your private way of letting things out. Expressing yourself and your feelings helps get through this a little easier.

11

Losing Friends to
Violence

by Daniel Navarro

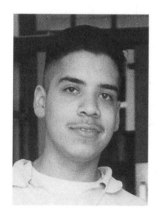

Maria Garcia, Parent-Student Advocate at Adamson High School in Dallas, Texas, introduced me to Daniel Navarro. He lost eight friends in four years to violence. Daniel is a quiet person whose sincerity stands out as you read his story. He is a senior at Adamson High School and will graduate in December.

Celebrating Cinco de Mayo in the park with my family when I was five was the first memory I ever had. I grew up in a family of four boys. I am the third child.

Between 1992 and 1995, I lost eight friends due mostly to gang activity. I lost my two best friends, Joe and Salvador.

Joe died when he was 15 years old. He carried a 9 millimeter gun that he always played with. For a joke, he would take the gun out and turn it backwards where it was pointing toward him. He was doing this at my friend's house when he accidentally pulled the trigger and shot himself in the face. Two of my friends were with him when this happened. One of them got to Joe, held him, and told him to wake up.

When I first heard about Joe's death, I couldn't believe it. Earlier that night, we tried to get him to go to a party with us, but he said, "Nah, just drop me off at home." So, we dropped him off and then we went to this party. I was using the phone when somebody told me, "Hey, Joe shot himself!"

The caller said, "He just shot himself at Enrique's house." I couldn't believe it. I miss Joe being here right now. He had already lost his dad and his mom and brother. Some times I think his life was so bad, he got careless.

Salvador was shot on October 19th. That was a horrible night. I was in a car and friends were in a van that was being chased by a white car. The car pulled up beside them and started shooting. We were behind a truck that was blocking our way and it wouldn't move. From the corner we saw the van going fast and the white car right behind them. In about two blocks we could hear gun shots. I looked at my home boy and said, "What happened?" he said, "I don't know. They probably shot at Sal and ..."

I went home and called Sal's house. His sister answered crying, and she said that everyone was at the hospital. I told her what happened. She said, "No, Salvador was in an accident." Then, I told her I would call her back later. When I called her back, her dad had told her that Sal was all right. I guess her dad didn't want to upset her by telling her the truth. When she told me that Sal was Okay, I went back to sleep. The next morning friends said, "Did you hear about Sal?" Then they said, "He's dead." We all cried together.

My other friends died because of car jackings and shootings that were gang related. Sometimes I think about my own life being in danger and sometimes I am scared. I try to deal with it by staying away from things that are about to happen. It's hard because when you see a friend getting beat up by someone, you can't just let him get beat up. You have to help him.

My brother, who used to be leader of a gang, has a job now and is doing well. With his encouragement, I plan on graduating, going to college, and majoring in architecture or business. He is always telling me to chill out and not be doing things. I tell others to keep away from gangs. Don't get in them. Watch out and be safe.

Words of Encouragement:

I have something to say to teenagers who have lost friends to violence. Think about the good times you had with your friends. Don't think about the bad times or how they got shot and all that because you will start to feel ugly. You will feel bad because you weren't there to help them and save them from what happened.

12

Grief From Losing Home & Security

by Blanca Martinez

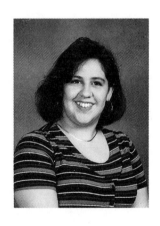

Many teenagers experience similar stages of grief when they have other kinds of significant losses. Blanca's story describes loss of her home to fire and her efforts to overcome her pain.

Blanca Martinez recently graduated from Sanger High after transferring from Lake Dallas High School. Her family is very close and at the end of her sophomore year, Blanca sang at a choir concert with her older brother, Conrado and older sister, Elizabeth. When she is not busy with school, athletics, or working, Blanca composes songs and writes poems. She plans to go to college.

When I think of "home," a lot of things come to my mind at once. Home is a place where you go to feel safe and secure. If you are sick, you go home. Being at home makes everything else seem okay.

I still remember the way my home was before it burned four years ago. My family had lived in the same house for 10 years. There were so many memories, everything we'd gone through, the good and the bad. We had many pictures of these times together.

I liked the house because it was comfortable. If it rained outside, I couldn't hear it. I felt safe. When I walked in the house at night, I wasn't afraid of anyone coming in. It was real comfortable.

Taquito was my pet parrot and he was very important to me. He would wake up the whole family early each morning by repeating, "Blanca, wake up!" He seemed to know my moods and if I started to cry, he would ask, "What's wrong?" He was always there.

When a person is secure with a home, they figure they'll always have it. But when tragedy strikes, and you lose your home, everything goes blank. You don't know where to go and you realize you don't own anything except for a car. This is hard thinking about this because it brings back memories. When my home burned, my family lost everything, including our pictures and Taquito.

It was second to the last period of the day at school and my brother, Conrado, came and got me out of class. He said something wrong had happened. Several things went through my mind. First, I thought my mom was hurt. Next, I thought about my dad. Then, I was afraid that someone was in the hospital.

As we walked down the hall, Conrado told me that our house was burning. I panicked. I thought, "Oh my God, my mother is there, or my sister is there and she is pregnant, oh my gosh!" I figured everyone was at home. My brother and I were both crying as we left school.

When we got to our neighborhood, we couldn't even make it to our home because there were too many ambulances and fire trucks blocking the street. Just as Conrado and I started running, I could see our mom running toward us crying. We couldn't say anything because it really hurt. We just stood there holding each other as we watched our house burn. I felt so helpless because there was nothing we could do. It was raining and our house continued to burn which seemed really odd to me. Then, I remembered my bird.

While standing there, I felt many different emotions. I was angry, scared, and nervous. I was nervous because I didn't know what was going to happen afterwards. I didn't know where we were going to go. I didn't know if we were going to stay in the same town or start over somewhere else. So many things went through my mind.

Later, I remember telling my father I was very angry. I asked, "Why does God have to take something away that you like so much? He's suppose to give you stuff you need."

After we saw our house burn, our family got separated. I don't know what happened during that time because I have forgotten. I don't remember where I went. I was totally out of it for about two weeks. I felt numb. I was told that a couple of days after the fire, my family checked into a hotel.

During that time a lot of people helped us out. They gave us food, money, and shelter. My friends were great. One friend named Chad knew how much I always worried about my hair, so he gave me a curling iron and brush. I felt so special. I didn't have to worry about things I needed because my friends were there.

Although I could depend on friends, I developed an overwhelming feeling of hopelessness. This feeling was mixed with feeling lonely. I didn't have anywhere to go. I didn't feel comfortable at the hotel, my aunt's or sister's. I got very sick and ended up in the hospital. After being released from the hospital, I developed new physical symptoms, all resulting from the traumatic experience.

As a family, this tragedy bonded us, we got closer. We became supportive for each other. My parents usually do not show emotion, but for something like this, they just opened up. We talked about the fire and what it had done to us.

I expressed my feelings during this hard time by singing and writing music. It helped me open up and describe what I was going through. Then one day it dawned on me that this horrible thing had happened, and I was going to have to get over it. The music gave me hope for a better future.

The past three months have been hard for me. My family moved from the town where I had gone to school for 13 years. And, last week, my brother, Conrado, left for the Marines in California. He is the first child in our family to move so far away. I hope it gets easier to accept because it sure is difficult to think about now!

Words of Encouragement: I would like to show my support to any teenager who has had a loss similar to mine by saying, "Cry all you want to. Sometimes things happen, but when there's something bad, eventually there's something good. There are many people who want to help. So allow them to do it."

13

Suggestions for Families

When you offer support to your grieving teenager, follow his or her lead, be patient, take it slowly, do not push. Your teenager may want you to be close-by although he or she may not feel like talking. Use this time to nurture, hold your teen and allow him or her the freedom to cry.

Eventually, your teenager may want to express reactions and concerns regarding the death. Demonstrate your love and respect by being attentive. Share what you know about getting through tough times. Tell about your past experiences of loss and what seemed to help you without trying to shift the focus to your needs. Your child will appreciate you and learn much.

Now is not the time to give a whole lot of advice or to make moralistic statements about the behavior of the person who died. Your teen is in a delicate emotional state, so choose arguments wisely and remember little things do not matter. You do not want to create more stress by arguing over trivial matters, like choice of clothing. Do not make an issue out of what your teenager wears during these days. Also, do not let your upset personal emotions have you make radical decisions at this time, like immediately removing all personal items of the deceased. Try instead to encourage quiet time where you can share good remembrances and low stress activities.

What to Say and What to Avoid Saying

Teenagers want to hear words they can relate to, and at the same time, words the other person truthfully feels. They want to hear something that is unique for them. Positive words of encouragement you might say are:

> "Do you want to talk about it?"
> "I know you're hurting. Can I hold you?"
> "I'd like to make it a quiet day. What would you
> like to do?"
> "Do you want to go to the funeral?"
> "It's normal to be angry when something like this
> happens. Do you want to go on a walk?"
> "It's always hard to understand when something that
> seems so unfair happens. Would you like to
> talk to a preacher, priest, rabbi or a
> counselor?"

Avoid making statements that discourage your teen from grieving or that place a time limitation on healing. **Do not say things like:**

> "How long are you going to keep on doing this?"
> "Go with things and make the best of it."
> "You've been grieving long enough, it's time to move
> on."

Memorials Help

Memorials help survivors remember their loved ones, and as you read the stories in this book, teenagers find that making memorials can be very comforting. Buying flowers, planting trees, donating money to a favorite cause, starting a fund in the person's name, recording a tape, writing poems, composing music, and making a scrapbook are beneficial activities that honor and celebrate the life of the person who died.

Some Decisions Have to be Made

Decisions have to be made during the first week of mourning regarding the funeral and burial. This is a difficult time because a bereaved person is extremely emotional and may be functioning on "autopilot" in order to get things done. Some people either lose their desire to care about what happens because of depression or they focus their energies on "micro-managing" the funeral and other arrangements. Because of the emotional nature of the time, it is recommended that major decisions, like giving away personal possessions of the deceased, selling the house and moving, quitting school, or changing jobs be made at a later date.

A teen's grieving family also may be thrown into unfamiliar or stressful new roles that require immediate decisions regarding the welfare of the family. If the parent who financially supports the family becomes ill or dies, monthly income may be interrupted which makes some families dependent on temporary outside sources. If this happens, there are community agencies available to help families. (Samples are found starting on page 84.)

Decisions Regarding Funeral and Burial

You may have to make decisions about the funeral or memorial service and burial. Use the funeral as a last loving gesture for the person who died. Pick out clothing with care for your loved one and select something the person liked. When deciding on clothing, music, verses, and parting words for the ceremony, you might want to choose a good mix between what the deceased person would want and what gives you peace.

After deciding on details for the funeral, including time and place, you also have to choose a place for burial. The fact that most people are mobile and move a lot makes this difficult. Do you bury your loved one close-by or a distance away where the rest of your relatives are buried? This is not an easy decision, but necessary.

Families also have to decide how they are going to tell their children about the death of a family member or close friend and determine how they are going to include their children in future activities regarding the funeral and burial. If you have younger children, you want to be honest with them from the very beginning about the cause of death and your feelings regarding your loss. Explain to them what to expect if and when they view the body before the funeral. Give details about the memorial service and let the choice be theirs' whether they want to go to the viewing and attend the funeral service. You may want to encourage their participation, but do not force it. Most counselors who work with grief, believe that children and teens heal better if they attend the funeral. If the person was killed in a bad accident, you may choose to keep the casket closed throughout all ceremonies.

During this time when you are struggling with making the "right" decisions, *remember,* people who heal best, work hard at keeping open conversation and positive memories about the deceased. Do not discourage people around you from discussing your loved one as this may be their best method for working through their upset feelings.

Decisions Regarding Personal Items of the Deceased

If they can, many people delay making the decision to go through personal items of the deceased. Going through and getting rid of personal affects may renew old memories and this might be very painful. Some people wait a year, others make the decision or are forced to do it sooner due to a move or other circumstance. Different family members will have different times when they want to do this. Each family member needs to have time alone to go through the room of the deceased and remember their loved one again by looking at what the person thought was special like clothing, personal affects, and correspondence. Afterwards, family members will have an idea what mementos would be special to them. More questions on this topic are answered at end of this book in the "Questions and Answers" section.

WARNING SIGNS: WHEN TO CALL FOR HELP

Depression for grief is natural. As the bereaved person works through months of pain and confusion, feelings of grief may come and go. There are occasions when laughter is welcomed and activities with friends become good experiences. Eventually, the grief depression slowly subsides and the person is free to concentrate on other areas of life while developing a positive attitude toward the future.

Suicide

As discussed earlier, suicide is a fear with teens, and families need to be watching for warning signs. When healing does not take place, depression may consume a person's life to the extent he or she withdraws from society or develops self-destructive behaviors. An isolated person may feel worthless, helpless, and become nonfunctional with thoughts of suicide. He or she may talk about suicide to friends. *These behaviors are serious; seek professional help.*

Disordered Eating

Another inappropriate or self-destructive behavior that may develop from lingering depression after a death is an eating disorder. Some teens focus on food either by compulsively overeating or drastically reducing the amount of food they eat. This is done in hopes they will divert or control everything unpleasant, including painful feelings of loss. Family members need to be concerned about their teenagers if they exhibit the following warning signs for eating disorders:

- Gain or lose 10 to 15 pounds in six weeks or less.
- Refuse to eat or won't eat when people are around.
- Obsess about weight and food.
- Believe in a distorted or unrealistic body image.
- Can't concentrate.
- Tired most of the time.
- Exhibit low self-esteem.
- Develop dental problems (bulimic) or respiratory and heart problems (anorexic) (16).

Call a counselor or physician to get referrals to qualified therapists or dietitians specialized in eating disorders. *Then call for an appointment.*

Inappropriate behaviors are used in several different ways to handle grief. These behaviors may appear in addition to other symptoms of depression or be the only symptoms to appear. An eating disorder presents one inappropriate behavior.

Drugs

Another inappropriate behavior that may exist to avoid facing grief is abuse of prescription or illegal drugs, or alcohol. Teenagers may feel they can dull their pain by using these drugs.

Sometimes it is difficult for parents to distinguish the difference between normal behavior for a teen or a teen who is using drugs. You can tell if your teen has a drug problem if you keep the communication open, stay alert to the activities and behavior of your teenager, and become familiar with the signs to help you identify a drug problem:

- Sudden, unexplained changes in behavior or mood that are extreme or that lasts for several days.
- Significant drop in grades or school performance.
- Loss of interests in school activities, sports, or hobbies.
- Rebellious attitude all of a sudden.
- Withdrawal from family.
- Drops old friends and is excessively influenced by new ones.
- Ignores personal grooming.
- Loss of weight; decrease in energy and drive.
- Change in sleep patterns.
- Signs of being secretive.
- Speaks with slurred speech or seems confused (17) .

If you suspect drug use, call your doctor or clinic to request a physical for your child in order to rule out any health problems. If your teen is using drugs, ask your doctor for referrals to psychologists and drug abuse counselors. There are also self-help groups, like Alcoholics Anonymous, social service agencies, drug treatment centers, school counselors, and listings in phone book under "drug abuse."

Other Risky Behaviors

Other inappropriate behaviors teenagers use to avoid coping with a death is their willingness to take life-threatening risks. Examples are reckless driving, practicing unprotected sex, crossing the street without looking, taking chances in sports, failing to protect self against crime, etc. When teens survive the risks they take, it relieves their stress level, but only temporarily (18). Although this behavior may be unintentional, it needs to be addressed by a grief counselor (See figure 13.1 for suggestions on how to help teens from developing risky behaviors).

TEEN ASSETS TO PROTECT FROM RISKY BEHAVIORS

Parents can help their teenagers by instilling the personal assets that keep them from risky behaviors. It is never too late to try to help your teens develop characteristics that make them strong.

Figure 13.1   TEEN ASSETS (19)

CATEGORY	PERSONAL ASSETS
Support	1. Family support
	2. Parent(s) as social source
	3. Parent communication
	4. Other adult resources
	5. Other adult communication
	6. Parent involvement in schooling
	7. Positive school climate
Parental Control	8. Consistent boundaries
	9. Even handed monitoring
	10. Fair discipline
	11. Time at home
	12. Positive peer influence

Structured Time Use	13. Involved in music
	14. Involved in school extra-curricular activities
	15. Involved in community organizations or activities
	16. Involved in church or synagogue
Educational Commitment	17. Achievement motivation
	18. Educational aspiration
	19. School performance
	20. Good use of homework
Positive Values	21. Values helping people
	22. Is concerned about world hunger
	23. Cares about people's feelings
	24. Values sexual restraint
Social Competence	25. Assertiveness skills
	26. Decision-making skills
	27. Friendship-making skills
	28. Planning skills
	29. Self-esteem
	30. Positive view of personal future

Establishing Open Conversation With Your Teen

When your teen is grieving may not be the best time to improve your relationship with him or her, but it may be the best opening you have had in years. Given the right circumstances, the time after the death of a loved one can be life changing. Figure 13.2 gives typical teen perspectives to help you understand your teen better.

The following are typical things that your teen might say to you if the conversation were open and flowing: (20)

- Be honest, I can spot a phony right away; the truth works best.
- Furnish me with guidelines; then I won't be testing the rules.
- Let me manage important parts of my life, as soon as I am able.
- Grant me privacy and time to myself, but still hug me often.
- Teach me living skills and encourage my creative side.
- Honor my feelings as they are neither right nor wrong.
- Show me that grief is normal when I lose something.
- Love me for who I am, not what you want me to be.
- Let me know you're not perfect, that you make mistakes, too.
- Seek my opinion; I have wisdom in many matters.

SERVICES TO HELP PEOPLE IN NEED

1. Interfaith Ministries or Christian Community Action

Telephone books or information operators will provide these local numbers or you may want to call a church or synagogue for referrals.

Most counties throughout the United States have an alliance of different churches that provide temporary assistance in the following areas: supplemental housing funds, emergency medication prescriptions, transportation for medical appointments and job interviews, limited utility assistance, clothing, and food.

2. United Way

Refer to your local directory for a telephone number. United Way provides an information and referral service to people inquiring about health and human services in their local communities.

3. Universities of higher learning are valuable sources that provide a variety of services for people in the community. Look in your telephone directory for phone numbers to those universities. Some of the services they provide are:

- Counseling for individuals, marriage, and family.
- Play therapy for children who have emotional problems.
- Diagnosis and treatment for children and teens who have reading, speech, hearing, or emotional problems.
- Tutoring for students who have learning problems.
- Financial assistance for college education.
- GED testing for residents who are 17 years old.
- Career planning and testing for those people wanting jobs.
- Dental assistance.
- Limited health services.
- Day care for preschoolers.

GRIEF RECOVERY OR SELF-HELP GROUPS

If you need grief recovery information or self-help groups in your area, you may want to consider the following sources:

1. Compassionate Friends
P.O. Box 3696, Oak Brook, IL 60522-3696
708/990-0010

This is a self-help group that provides information and connects grieving parents and siblings to support groups throughout the United States.

2. The National Hospice Organization
1901 North Moore St., Suite 901, Arlington, VA 22209
703/243-5900
Web Site: WWW.NHO.ORG
Upon request, this organization will provide you with a directory of hospices in the United States.

3. National Self-Help Clearinghouse
25 West 43rd Street, Suite 620, New York, NY 10036
212/354-8525   Fax: 704 6759687
Web Site: SELFHELPWEB.ORG
This organization provides names of different support groups in your area.

4. Compassion Books
477 Hannah Branch Road, Burnsville, NC 28714
704/675-5909
Contact Compassion Books for publications and other resources on coping and grief recovery.

5. Survivors of Suicide
P.O. Box 1353, Dayton, OH 45401-1932
973/297-9096 or 973/297-4777

6. Twinless Twins Support Group, International
Dr. Raymond W. Brandt, Director
11220 St. Joe Road, Ft. Wayne, IN 46835-9737
219/627-5414
Web Site: WWW.WI.COM-TWINLESS
email: BRANDT MAIL.FWI.COM

This organization will furnish names of support groups throughout the United States for twins who have lost their twin. There is also a Twins World magazine, Twinless Times publication, and books you can order by writing or calling.

7. Grief Recovery Hotline
1-800-445-4808

If you need immediate help and want to talk to someone who is trained in grief counseling call this number.

Getting Information and Help for An Eating Disorder

Call a counselor or physician to get referrals to qualified therapists or dietitian specialist if you suspect your teenager has an eating disorder. Then, call for an appointment. If you need information on self-help groups in your area for eating disorders, call or write the following sources.

1. ANAD-National Association of Anorexia Nervosa and Associated Disorders
Box 7, Highland Park, IL 60035

2. American Anorexia/Bulimia Association
418 E.76th Street, New York, NY 10021
212/734-1114

3. Anorexia Nervosa and Related Eating Disorders
P.O. Box 5102, Eugene, OR 97405

4. Consumer Information Center
Department 551A, Pueblo, CO 81009
Write for pamphlet: "Eating Disorders"

5. American Academy of Child & Adolescent Psychiatry
3615 Wisconsin Avenue, NW, Washington, DC 20016
        Send self-addressed, stamped business-size envelope for
a fact sheet: "Teenagers with Eating Disorders."

6. American Psychiatric Association: Div. of Public Affairs
1400 K St. NW, Washington, DC 20005
        Send self-addressed, stamped business-size envelope for
booklet: "Let's talk Facts About Eating Disorders."

7. National Institute of Child Health & Human Development
P.O. Box 29111, Washington, DC 20040
        Write for pamphlet: "Facts About Anorexia Nervosa."

8. National Mental Health Association
1021 Prince Street, Alexandria, VA 22314
        Write for fact sheet: "Anorexia and Bulimia."

Getting Information and Help for Drug Use

        If you need information on self-help groups in your
area for teenage drug abuse, call or write the following
sources:

1. Al-Anon Family Group Headquarters
        See your telephone white pages. Resource for family
members and friends of alcoholics. Free, nonprofessional,
worldwide organization.

2. National Families in Action (drug prevention materials
        and information)
2296 Henderson Mill Road, Suite 300, Atlanta, GA 30345
770-934-6364   fax 770-934-7137

This agency publishes, Drug Abuse Update, a quarterly journal of news and information on drug prevention. Cost: $25 for four issues.

3. Hazelden Foundation
Pleasant Valley Road, Box 176, Center City, MN 55012
1-800-328-9000

This foundations supplies educational materials and self-help literature for participants in 12-step recovery programs.

4. Nar-Anon Family Group Headquarters
P.O. Box 2562, Palos Verdes Peninsula, CA 90274
310-547-5800

This organization supports people who have friends or family members with drug problems.

5. National Clearinghouse for Alcohol & Drug Information
Box 2345, Rockville, MD 20852
1-800-SAY-NOTO or 301/468-2600

Call for information on alcohol and drug abuse.

6. National Council on Alcoholism, Inc.
12 West 21st Street, New York, NY 10010
212/206-6770

Provides information about alcoholism and alcohol problems.

14

Suggestions for Friends

The Miracle of Friendship

There's a miracle called friendship
that dwells within the heart
and you don't know how it happens
or where it gets its start.
But the happiness it brings you
always gives a special lift,
and you realize that friendship
is God's most precious gift.

Copyright J Mar

HELPING A FRIEND THROUGH GRIEF
by Donna O' Toole, M.A.

1. Be There for Them

Grieving people need support and presence much
more than advice. It is important to offer support
over time.

2. Initiate and Anticipate

Grieving people often don't know or can't ask for what they need. Suggest times you'll be with them. Tell them ways you'd like to help.

3. Listen

It's often hard to believe a loss has really happened. Grieving people often need to talk about it a lot and tell the stories over and over. Listening without judgment or interruption can be the most important gift you can give.

4. Avoid clichés and Easy Answers

"I care"..."You're in my thoughts" or "I'm with you" may be the best response.

5. Silence is Golden

Sometimes there are no words for grief and no words that bring enough comfort to take away the pain. Silence can demonstrate your trust and acceptance.

6. Accept and Encourage the Expression of Feelings

Reassure the person that grief has many feelings... that feelings are like barometers that indicate our internal weather. Expressing feelings can help change the weather. Suggest non-hurtful ways. (Cry, punch bag, go running, etc.)

7. Offer Opportunities and Safety for Remembering

There are many times during grief that remembering helps the healing and growth process. Offer to revisit places and people who can help them get their questions answered or remember and can confirm the importance of the loss.

8. **Learn About the Grief Process**

   It will help with your fears and feelings of helplessness. When appropriate, share this with your friend as a natural process.

9. **Help the Person Find Support and Encouragement**

   Help your friend find a variety of supports to deal with different feelings and needs.

10. **Allow the Person to Grieve at His or Her Own Pace**

    Grief is an individual process. Your ability to not judge the length of time it takes will lighten the pressure to conform to other peoples' needs or ways, and will enhance self-trust.

11. **Be Patient...**

    With yourself and your friend. You may need to give more of yourself than you imagined. Make sure you have your own means of support and self-care to see you through.

12. **Provide for Times of Lightheartedness**

    Grief can be like swimming upstream...sometimes you need to get out of it and recoup. Laughter and play are wonderful ways to regain some needed energy.

13. **Believe in the Person's Ability to Recover and Grow**

    Your hope and faith may be needed when theirs fails. Your trust in the other's ability to heal is essential. Listen and be with them in emotional pain. DON'T PUSH.

15

Suggestions for School Counselors

PREPARE FOR A CRISIS

The best time to plan bereavement support for teenagers at school is before a crisis. Detailed plans are impossible because each case is unique and requires different techniques, but it helps if counselors know some of the logistics, like who is available if more counselors are needed and what rooms can be used for small groups.

It is also good for counselors to prepare the school staff for a loss before it happens. Arrange to speak at the beginning of the school year at an in-service workshop or provide a brief paper on grief information for the teachers. They need to be informed about the teenage issues related to loss, death, and grief. If teachers and principals are informed about possible behavioral changes in students who have losses, they will understand what these students are experiencing and provide support if needed (21).

When a death involves one or more students, counselors need to speak to each classroom briefly, answer any questions the teenagers might have, and take upset students with them to different locations in order to have small groups.

Counselors may end up having several ad hoc groups that give the students an opportunity to express their emotions, discuss the cause of death, remember their friend or friends who died, and decide what they can do to help the grieving family. During this time, some students may have emotions that remind them of other losses. They will need to discuss these issues with a counselor individually.

Counselors should plan to be available each morning before school and during the day for those students who want to visit. In time, counselors can make decisions regarding ongoing small groups for grief counseling and individual counseling for those who need help with their bereavement.

Activities for Individual or Group Counseling

- Journal—Encourage your grieving teens to keep journals and write about their losses. They can write about who they lost and why they miss them. Most people can express themselves by writing, but find it difficult to verbally discuss how they feel. This exercise helps them process through their pain, accept their loss, and heal.

- My Story—Writing for this activity will require a suggested outline for the young person to follow. Counselors may want to work with this activity in small segments. After the student completes a section, discuss what has been written. Ask questions about the person who died and ask about feelings. It is an excellent method for processing through a loss and can be used for groups or individually. When this project is completed, most students want to keep a printed copy. This is the outline the kids in this book used and it worked well.

My Story

I. Your Personal Background
    A. Your First Memory
    B. First Birthday You Can Remember
    C. Your Favorite Safe Place As A Kid
    D. Family Trips

II. Relationship With Person Who Died
    A. First Memory You Have Of This Person
    B. Favorite Thing Person Did for You
    C. Favorite Activities You Did Together
    D. Funny Things You Did Together

III. Person Who Died
    A. Funny Things He or She Did
    B. Things Person Did That Annoyed You
    C. How This Person Encouraged or
       Influenced You

IV. Loss
    A. Cause of death
    B. Emotional Reactions

V. Ways You Deal With Grief That Are Helpful
    A. Resources of Support
    B. Family Rituals To Remember Person
    C. Your Favorite Safe Place Now
    D. Recommendations for Teens With Losses

VI. Personal Memorials
    A. Drawings
    B. Poems
    C. Original Music
    D. Other Ideas

- Letters—Many grieving teens like to write letters to their loved ones to tell them about daily activities. This provides comfort and allows them time to accept their loss. It also provides an opportunity for the teen to say things they did not get to say before the death.
- Collages—Teenagers can decorate a box to place small personal items of the deceased. They may want to use several old photographs and make a collage. This provides something concrete for the grieving teen to hold, look at, and remember.
- Poems—Poems allow self-expression. Teens should be encouraged to compose original poems regarding their feelings and loss. If teens do not want to write their own poems, have them look for poems that represent the way they feel. Encourage the teenagers to read their poems aloud and discuss feelings.
- Music—Teenagers select music that identifies their problems. Have them bring CD's or audio tapes to counseling sessions and discuss the words and music. This activity allows them to get in touch with their feelings.
- Scrapbooks—If there are personal items or plenty of photographs of the person who died, have the teens organize scrapbooks to preserve those cherished memories. Teens will get great pleasure from sharing completed scrapbooks with their family and friends.
- Bibliotheraphy—Use fiction or nonfiction to help teenagers cope with their losses. Read and discuss a book or short stories so they can identify with the character or characters they read about. This also provides a way they can express reactions to grief and learn that their feelings are natural. Examples of books to use for bibliotherapy are: (22)

Bridge to Terabithia (Paterson 1977)
The Fall of Freddie the Leaf (Buscaglia 1982)
Shira: A Legacy of Courage (Grollman 1988)
Tiger Eyes (Blume 1981)

Long-Term Follow-Up

Holidays, birthdays, and anniversaries are difficult and teenagers seldom forget these dates. It is impossible for counselors to remember so many different days, but the one year anniversaries of death need to be documented in order to help each grieving teen get through that particular day. Ask each teen how he or she would like to spend the time with you. A card with a short message may be enough, but you might also want to be creative and think of something else special to do to honor the young person's feelings and memory of his or her loved one.

It is hard to plan a closing session for grief counseling because teens have emotions that come and go. Slowly, they stop asking for appointments and the counselor sees less and less of them. In time, counselors know these teens have reached a point where they feel confident and strong enough to independently move forward on their own.

16

Common Questions Teenagers Ask

Death robs us of our loved ones and leaves us with intense pain. During this time, when we feel confused, important decisions have to be made. The choices are easier to manage if we are provided some direction. Hopefully, the following questions and answers will help you.

Question: My grandmother is in the hospital dying with cancer. She is medicated and on several monitors but remains coherent enough to visit with the family. I cannot bear to see her suffer and have tried to tell her that I wish I could do something to relieve her pain. Although I want her to know how I feel, the words won't come out, and then I lose my nerve. What can I do?

Answer: Write your grandmother a letter and express your feelings. Tell her how much you love her. Think of anything else you want her to know because this might be your last opportunity. Also, consider including a poem written by you or one that appeals to you. If you cannot verbally express what you have written, read it to her or have someone else read it while you are there or visit her soon after.

Question: My friend died and I want to go to the funeral. I have never been to a funeral before and don't know what to expect. What do I do? Will they allow me to see my friend?

Answer: Memorial traditions vary among different ethnic groups and cultures (see pages 107-108). In most cases, the family makes decisions regarding the funeral service. Find out what funeral home is helping your friend's family. Call and find out if you can view the body before the service and when, and take a parent or a close friend. Be aware this is a serious time to show respect. Most people say a silent prayer. Do not stay too long, there are those who want to be alone. You will also have an opportunity to attend the service. Wear good clothes to the funeral, which may be at the funeral home or at a religious place of worship. At the service, some families have the casket opened, others choose to have a closed casket. The minister, rabbi, or priest, will speak about your friend and conclude with a parting message. Some families also speak or read poems. Usually there are a couple of songs. The whole service lasts less than an hour. It is a good time to cry, to remember, and to say good-bye. The service at the cemetery allows people to realize the finality of the death. Family and friends often take individual roses or flowers to leave on the casket. It symbolizes their love.

Question: My friend committed suicide. Several of us feel like we should have recognized his depression and done something to prevent this senseless death. We all feel horrible. Boy did we ever mess up!

Answer: Sometimes people are experts at concealing their true feelings. It is difficult to recognize the threat of suicide. All of you may have done the best with what you knew. Know now that the decision to die was his, not yours. You cannot control the actions of others. Continue to talk with your friends. Discuss these issues, help each other understand, and try to lose the guilt.

Question: My best friend was just killed in a drive by shooting. He was an innocent by-stander. I have never lost any other family member or friend and I don't think I'm getting over the grief. Will it always hurt this much? What can I do to make it better?

Answer: There is no set time for grieving to end. Healing from a death of a loved one improves with time and takes a great deal of work. It is a process by which you can proceed step by step (See chapter 14). You may need someone to guide you along the way so you can start healing, like a school counselor or minister. You will never totally forget, but in time you will remember the happy times as you move on with your life.

Question: My best friend, Shane, died two weeks ago. It's been really hard. All of my friends have been great, but I have a problem. They have the best intentions, but my friends won't leave me alone, especially the girls. They cry whenever they see me and put their arms around my neck, shoulders, and pat my back. It is constant. At the funeral home I did not get time alone with my best friend because there were at least four of them hanging on me constantly. I don't want to sound ungrateful because I do need their friendship. I'd just like my space some of the time. How do I get them to back off without making them mad? I don't think I can tell them.

Answer: Your friends are sharing your pain and have no idea they are going to extremes or that you need personal space. Speak with the school counselor and explain your situation. This professional can speak to several of the girls and invite them to a grief support group. The counselor can explain you need a break. I know your friends will understand and will follow through with the recommended suggestions. Then, you can reach out when you are ready. Sometimes teenagers need directions on how to react and help friends who grieve.

Question: I have to decide who I want to live with. Mom was killed in a car accident last month. I can live with my step-dad, who I live with now, or my grandmother, who lives in another state, or my older sister who lives in an apartment in a near-by town. My step-dad said I could continue to live here, but I don't know what to do. School won't be out for another five months. There are too many decisions. I'm really confused. What should I do?

Answer: Death has brought major changes to your life. If your mom died last month, you are still trying to deal with your emotions. Do not make any major decisions right now, like where to live permanently if you do not have to. Give yourself some time. If no one is rushing you to move, stay in school and take the time to get over some of your pain. Then, break down this huge picture and deal with it in small segments. Think of it as a puzzle, it will be much easier. After following these suggestions and reading this book, you will be able to evaluate and weigh all the options.

Question: When my dad died a month ago, my close friends suddenly disappeared. After the funeral, they quit calling me or coming by. I have so much to deal with, I don't think I can take much more. Why are they doing this to me?

Answer: I don't think your friends intentionally planned on hurting you. Often middle school kids do not know what to say to a friend who has suffered a loss. They feel awkward and are afraid of making an uncomfortable situation worse, so they avoid contact. Give it a month or two and they'll start including you again. I'm more concerned about the other problems that you failed to explain. Please talk with your mom or care provider, and think about visiting a professional counselor. It sounds like you may need some help to get through this tough time.

Question: Ever since Mom died, I have worn her jewelry and some of her clothes. I don't need the clothes, but like to wear them because they were her's. My friends found out I was wearing Mom's sweaters and freaked out. They couldn't believe I would want to do such a thing. Am I weird or something?

Answer: No, you are not weird. The jewelry is a wonderful reminder of your mom, and you might want to hold a few pieces for keepsakes. Some people feel at peace when wearing clothing of their loved ones. You do what is right for you. Explain to your friends that the jewelry and clothes give comfort. If they continue to give you a hard time and make you feel weird, consider limiting your time with them.

Question: It's been less than a year since Dad died unexpectedly with a heart attack. I'm having a rough time dealing with feelings. It started when I found out that he died. Instead of crying, I was mad at him! The anger has intensified. I'm a terrible person to be around. Yesterday, I punched my fist through my car that Dad helped me buy. This is driving me crazy. He was a great father. Why am I so mad at him?

Answer: It sounds like you and your dad had a close relationship. I imagine he supported you in many ways. It is normal to feel mad. Although you know your father did not choose to die, you feel like he chose to leave you. You may feel like he abandoned you. Know that you are mad at your loss and not at your dad. Your dad was taken at a time when you need him the most. Don't be hard on yourself. If you haven't already done it, feel free to cry. In time, start concentrating on the positive. What would your dad want you to do? Remember some of your plans for your future and follow through as much as possible. Remember the good times. Also, you might want to think of some type of memorial you can make that has significance for you. To relieve the stress and anger, exert energy each day. Jogging is excellent.

Question: My sister, a year younger than me, was killed in a car wreck her sophomore year in high school. It has been eight months since her death. My dad has been cleaning my sister's room and throwing away many items. He has even taken down photographs of my sister. I'm furious! It is as though my sister never existed. Every time I tell my dad to leave my sister's things alone, we end up yelling at each other. How can I make him leave things as they were?

Answer: You and your dad have chosen two different ways to deal with your sister's death. Unfortunately, they are in conflict with each other and will only cause more heartache. It might help you to understand that your resistance to change is your attempt to hold on to your sister and your dad may be trying to remove his pain by getting rid of your sister's personal items. You need a third party to help resolve some of these issues. Perhaps your mom? What does she want? Do you have a grandmother or an aunt, uncle, or older cousin you can call for help with this issue? Have them encourage your dad to join a grief group that periodically includes family members. Also, you would benefit from a teenage grief group. Ask your school counselor to make recommendations. Continue to talk to your dad about topics that don't cause arguments. Remember, you need each other!

Question: My dad was killed in a car wreck last year. It was so unfair because he was only 36. Now, I have my older brother and Mother. I am very insecure. Sometimes I panic because I'm afraid of losing one of them. I don't think I could survive that. What can I do? I can't go everywhere they go.

Answer: "Why's" are almost always impossible to answer in a situation like yours. Instead of trying to understand why this happened to your dad, concentrate on what you can do to work through your grief so that you will become stronger. Your fear of losing another family member is understandable and you have done well to identify the problem. Join a teenage grief group where you'll find support from peers who know what you are experiencing and can be there for you. The planned activities will also help you process your grief. Within five to six months you should be able to concentrate on other areas of your life and start thinking about your future. If the panic feelings are persistent or return after group counseling, seek individual counseling.

Question: My older brother, who is out of school, never got along very well with Mom. Before Mom died, she was in the hospital for a week. He never came to visit her. After she died, he refused to talk about her or about their relationship. He is still bitter. How can I make him get help?

Answer: You can't force your brother to get help. He is the one who must evaluate his situation and determine if he wants to reach out for family support or professional help. You can let him know that you love him and that you'll be there if he should need you.

FUNERAL TRADITIONS

Buddism is the fourth largest religion in the world, originating in India and most common in Asia, but it is Great Britain's fastest growing religion. Buddha preached that existence is a continuing cycle of death and rebirth. Good deeds are rewarded in the next life and evil deeds are punished with sickness and misfortune. When a person dies, a monk is summoned to recite special sermons and the sutra (scripture) of the dead. The monk then applies the "last water" to the lips of the deceased, after which the body is bathed and properly dressed. A funeral ceremony follows where the mourners speak to honor the deceased. The person is then cremated. Death rites commonly continue for a number of days with the bereaved family hosting meals (23).

Traditional Jews believe the dead person's body is a shell that no longer holds the soul. The person's body is ceremoniously cleasned (Chevar Chedush), but not embalmed. Therefore, burial must take place within 24 hours. The person's body is wrapped in a shroud to show the person came into the world with nothing and is leaving with nothing. The casket is wooden so that it will decay (dust to dust). The funeral ceremony is rather short with a symbolic piece of ribbon or clothing being torn to signify a torn heart. The immediate family dedicates an entire week to the memory of their loved one; they do not cook as food is brought in by friends and relatives. They cry as much as they can and remember the fun times with that person. This allows them to move forward (8).

    Muslims teach that life has a purpose and ends in death. Death and dying are discussed often by families. At the time of death, people weep freely and pray with a religious leader to ask God for forgiveness. They believe that weeping freely releases sorrow. As with the Jews, the person's body is bathed with women washing women and men washing men. The body is usually wrapped in white cotton cloth. A woman's face is covered and only seen by family; a man's face is only seen by family and friends. Bodies are not embalmed, and have to be buried within 24 hours, but without a casket. After 3-7 days of mourning, the family often returns to work and normal routines.

    Within the **Protestant** religion, there are many different denominations with many ethnic and cultural backgrounds. Most Protestants believe in eternal life and that after death they will be reunited with their loved ones. Typical Protestant rituals were mentioned on page 102, people gather for visitation and then a funeral or memorial service. The person's body is usually embalmed, so the burial may not take place for 3-5 days, until all the family can be present. Often an ornate casket and flower bouquets are used by the bereaved family and friends to show respect. Neighbors and friends may provide meals for a few days. After the funeral service, family members meet and renew acquaintances. They return to former routines as they are emotionally able.

    Catholics believe that Jesus promises the believer life in heaven with Him, but if the person was bad he may go to Hell or somewhere in between, Purgatory. There are two funeral services: rosary mass, a series of prayers for the family, friends, and the deceased, and then a funeral mass, which is said as a celebration into eternal life. A priest leads both masses. Many symbols connect spiritual beliefs to give comfort and are used during the funeral rites.

Recommended Reading for Teenagers

Bode J. *Death Is Hard to Live With.* New York: Delacorte Press; 1993.

Buscaglia L. *The Fall of Freddie the Leaf.* New York: Holt & Co.; 1982.

Case BJ. *Living Without Your Twin.* Portland, OR: Tibbutt Publishers; 1993.

Gaffron N. *Dealing With Death.* San Diego, CA: Lucent Books; 1989.

Gootman M. *When A Friend Dies.* Minneapolis, MN: Free Spirit; 1994.

Grollman EA. *Straight Talk About Death for Teenagers.* Boston, MA: Beacon Press; 1993.

Hagaard ME. *Coping With Death and Grief.* Minneapolis, MN: Lerner Publications; 1990.

Lemiux CM. *Coping With The Loss of a Pet.* Reading, PA: Wallace Clark Publishers; 1992.

Recommended Reading for Professionals

Boyd-Franklin N, Steiner GL, Boland MG (Eds.). *Children, Families, and HIV/ AIDS.* New York: Guilford Press; 1995.

Capuzzi D. *Suicide Prevention in the Schools: Guidelines for Middle and High School Settings.* Alexandra, Virginia: American Counseling Assn.; 1994.

Cook AS. *Helping the Bereaved: Therapeutic Interventions for Children, Adolescents, and Adults.* New York: Basic Books; 1992.

Goldstein AP, Huff C (Eds.). *The Gang Intervention Handbook.* Research press available through American Counseling Assn, Alexandria, VA; (1993).

Grollman EA (Ed.). *Bereaved Children & Teens.* Boston: Beacon Press; 1995.

Oats M. *Death in the School Community.* Alexandra, Virginia: American Counseling Assn.; 1993.

Oaklander V. *Windows to Our Children.* Highland, NY Center for Gestalt Development; 1988.

Rosen H. *Unspoken Grief.* Rutgers: The State University of New Jersey; 1990.

Tatelbaum J. *The Courage To Grieve.* New York: Harper & Row; 1980.

Webb NB (Ed.). *Helping Bereaved Children.* New York: Guilford Publications; 1993.

Book References

1. Conference on *Forum for Death Education and Counseling*; 1981.
2. Erickson E. *Youth and Crises*. New York: Norton; 1968.
3. Rosenberg HM, Ventura SJ, Maurer JD, et al. *Births & Deaths: U. S. 1995*. Monthly vital statistics report; v. 45 No. 3, supp. 2, p. 31. Hyattsville, Maryland: National Center for Health Statistics.
4. Corr CA. Entering Into Adolescent Understanding of Death. In E.A. Grollman (Ed.), *Bereaved Children and Teens* p.21-35. Boston: Beacon Press; 1995.
5. Wendel P. Counselors' Role in Youth Gang Prevention and Intervention. *Counseling Today*. 1997: v.39, p.1; 10-11; 16-17.
6. Malley PB, Kush G, Bogo RJ. School-Based Suicide Prevention and Intervention Programs. *Prevention Research*. 1996: v. 3, p. 9-11.
7. Henry CS. A Human Ecological Approach To Adolescent Suicide. *Prevention Research*. 1996: v.3, p. 1-5.
8. Wartik N. Learning To Mourn. *American Health*. 1996: p. 76-96.
9. Irish DP. Children & Death: Diversity in Universality. In EA. Grollman (Ed.). *Bereaved Children and Teens*. 1995: p. 77-91.
10. O'Toole D. When Grief Doesn't Heal. In *Growing Through Grief*. Burnsville, NC: Mountain Rainbow Publications. 1989: p.300.
11. Tatelbaum J. *The Courage To Grieve*. New York: Harper & Row; 1980.
12. Harris ES. Adolescent Bereavement Following the Death of a Parent: An Exploratory Study. *Child Psychiatry & Human Development*. 1991:v.21 (4) p. 267-281.
13. Hogan N, DeSantis L. Adolescent Sibling Bereavement: An Ongoing Attachment. Qualitative Health Research. 1992: v.2 (2) p.159-177.
14. Glass JC. Death, Loss, & Grief in High School Students. The High School Journal. Feb./Mar. The University of North Carolina Press; 1990.
15. Ibid
16. Arbetter S. The A's & B's of Eating Disorders. *Current Health 2*. Sept. 1994: p.6-12.
17. U.S. Department of Education. Growing Up Drug Free: Parent's Guide to Prevention, Washington, D.C.
18. Stevenson RG. "I Thought About Death All the Time...": Students, Teachers, and the Understanding of Death. In EA Grollman (Ed.). *Bereaved Children & Teens*. Boston: Beacon Press. 1995: p. 181-194.
19. *Personal Assets That Protect Youth From Risky Behavior*. Training Session; 1996.
20. Rhea G, Murphy A. *What Your Child Might Say...* Workshop handout.
21. Glass JC. Death, Loss, & Grief in High School Students. *The High School Journal*. Feb/March. University of North Carolina Press; 1990.
22. Corr CA. Entering Into Adolescent Understanding of Death. In EA. Grollman (Ed.). *Bereaved Children & Teens*. Boston: Beacon Press; 1995; p. 21-35.
23. Wangu MB. *Buddhism: World Religions*. New York, NY: Facts on File, Inc.; 1993.
24. McLaughlin MA. Life, Death, & the Catholic Child. In E.A. Grollman (Ed.). *Bereaved Children and Teens*. 1995: p. 129-140.

"There is a Wholeness..."

For my sermon on the first Yom Kippur after my son Aaron's death I took my text from The Missing Piece, a children's book by Shel Silverstein. It is a story about a circle from which a large triangular wedge had been cut. The circle wanted to be whole, so it went looking for the missing piece. But because it was incomplete, it could only roll slowly. It admired the flowers along the way. It chatted with butterflies. It enjoyed the sunshine.

It found lots of pieces, but none fit. So it left them all by the side of the road and kept on searching. Then one day it found a piece that fit exactly. It was so happy. Now it could be whole, with nothing missing. But as a perfect circle, it rolled too fast to notice the flowers or talk to the butterflies. When it realized how different the world seemed, it stopped, left its missing piece by the side of the road and rolled on-appreciating life again.

I suggested in my sermon that in some strange sense we are more whole when we are incomplete. The man who has everything is in some ways a poor man. He will never know what it feels like to yearn, to hope, to dream. He will never know the experience of getting something he has always wanted and never had.

There is a wholeness about a person who can give his time, his money, his strength, to others and not feel diminished. There is a wholeness about the person who has come to terms with his limitations, who knows who he is and what he can and cannot do. There is a wholeness about the man or woman who has learned he or she is strong enough to go through a tragedy and survive, the person who can lose someone through death, through estrangement, and still feel complete. at that point nothing can scare you. You have been through the worst and come through it whole.